The Green Smoothie
Bible

The Green Smoothie

Bible

Super-Nutritious Drinks to Lose Weight, Boost Energy and Feel Great

KRISTINE MILES

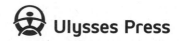 Ulysses Press

Published in the U.S. by
ULYSSES PRESS
P.O. Box 3440
Berkeley, CA 94703
www.ulyssespress.com

ISBN13: 978-1-56975-974-5
Library of Congress Control Number 2011926023

Acquisitions Editor: Keith Riegert
Managing Editor: Claire Chun
Editors: Lauren Harrison, Susan Lang
Production: Judith Metzener
Front cover design: what!design @ whatweb.com
Cover photo: © ma-k/istockphoto.com

Printed in United States by Bang Printing

10 9 8 7 6

Distributed by Publishers Group West

NOTE TO READERS
This book has been written and published strictly for informational and educational purposes only. It is not intended to serve as medical advice or to be any form of medical treatment. You should always consult your physician before altering or changing any aspect of your medical treatment and/or undertaking a diet regimen, including the guidelines as described in this book. Do not stop or change any prescription medications without the guidance and advice of your physician. Any use of the information in this book is made on the reader's good judgment after consulting with his or her physician and is the reader's sole responsibility. This book is not intended to diagnose or treat any medical condition and is not a substitute for a physician.

Contents

PART TWO
Green Smoothie Recipes

Introduction

While visiting a girlfriend in the United Kingdom last year, I made a green smoothie for her 18-month-old daughter. Little Alice was fascinated by the whirring of the blender and the evolving bright green liquid. I placed a small cup in her willing hands, and as she tasted the smooth green liquid for the very first time, she relished it—and so did much of her face.

I wasn't lucky enough to discover green smoothies at 18 months of age, but I believe I reached a high point in my digestively challenged journey at 33 years. In seeking improved health and well-being, I read many books, researched online, visited health professionals, experimented with different ways of eating, and experienced many "aha!" moments along the way. I removed wheat and dairy from my diet, and ultimately all gluten-containing foods, got rid of coffee, reduced the amount of sugar, returned to a vegetarian diet, discovered raw foods, and finally came upon green smoothies!

I lead a busy life as a full-time physiotherapist along with running two other home-based businesses, writing, and being a wife to my best friend, Ben. People ask me where I get my energy and I believe it's partly attitude, as I am a persistent, committed, and optimistic person. I also eat a clean, unprocessed diet. I don't consume foods that disagree with me, I eat a high proportion of raw plant-based foods, and I drink a green smoothie every morning without fail. Whether I am up early or late, traveling or at home, a green smoothie is a must for me as it is for my husband. Just 16 ounces or 2 cups (500 mL) sees me through to lunchtime with ease, with no blood sugar dips. It's easy to digest in the morning and so very convenient. In 3 to 4 minutes I have a smoothie prepped and made, and the blender cleaned, and if I am in a hurry, the smoothie is easy to transport to work in a glass jar.

In 2007 I built a website devoted to green smoothies. What started as an opportunity to share what I had learned, and to post some of my favorite recipes and photos, became a much bigger deal, with thousands of hits and wonderfully supportive feedback from people ranging from novices to experienced green smoothie drinkers. Now I am thrilled and so very grateful to turn my passion and hobby into *The Green Smoothie Bible*, which contains everything you need to know about green smoothies, including what they are, how they benefit your body, and, of course, all the recipes you need to get going.

Warm and green regards,
Kristine Miles

PART ONE

About Green Smoothies

What Are Green Smoothies?

A green smoothie is a fruit smoothie with raw leafy greens blended through it so that it tastes like fruit but looks green. Although greens are incredibly nutritious, many people struggle to eat enough of them. Adding fruit makes the greens taste great and is also a clever way of getting more fruit into a diet. Some people lack both fruit and greens in their diets, and green smoothies are a delicious way to fulfill both needs.

People who have introduced green smoothies into their diets report many health benefits such as clearer skin, improved digestion, weight loss, and better mood. Those following a raw food diet have especially embraced this nutritional powerhouse to boost an already nutritious diet, often finding some missing element that helps them achieve excellent health and vitality.

What Goes into a Green Smoothie?

I have to start by saying that green smoothies don't taste horrible! Although they are green, they taste like the fruit in them. Obviously, if you go overboard with greens, the smoothie will taste like the greens in it, but generally you don't taste the greens much, if at all. The green smoothies in this book are raw and mostly vegan, meaning no cooked or pasteurized ingredients and no dairy products, which are the base of traditional smoothies. This means no recipe uses cow, goat, or sheep milk or yogurt, nor any pasteurized milks such as soy, rice, or oat. As alternatives to water, only non-heat-treated, plant-based milks made from raw nuts and seeds are used in these recipes. When I say mostly vegan it is because some of my recipes do contain bee products such as pollen and honey. These are optional, of course.

Generally, I recommend using 40 percent greens and 60 percent fruit. For beginners, start with about 10 percent and gradually increase over time. If you do happen to overdo the greens, try some sweetener, a bit of vanilla, or some lemon juice to take the edge off.

How to Make a Green Smoothie

Making a green smoothie couldn't be easier. All you do is put greens, roughly chopped fruit, and liquid (usually water) in a blender and blend for 1 to 2 minutes. It doesn't matter in what order you add the ingredients (I put the liquid and solids in at the same time). If the recipe calls for water, ideally use filtered or pure spring water. Some recipes call for juice, nut milk, or herbal tea as the liquid base. Always blend the ingredients thoroughly to break up and incorporate the greens. Serves 2.

BEGINNER'S RECIPE
    3 to 4 ripe bananas
    1 teaspoon vanilla extract
    2 cups water
    handful of fresh, clean spinach

All recipes in this book make around 1 quart (1 liter), enough to fill two large glasses each holding 2 cups (500 mL) of green smoothie.

I am a fan of using as few ingredients as possible so I can actually taste what's in the smoothie. Combine six different fruits if you like, but the result is usually a smoothie with an ill-defined and uninspiring flavor. For instance, you will taste both banana and berries in a banana-berry smoothie, but add apple, pear, and peach and the smoothie gets very confused.

My best advice is to use ingredients that you enjoy eating; otherwise you will be less inclined to drink them. Just because you are drinking something extremely healthy does not mean it can't taste great. When inventing your own concoctions, you're bound to have the odd failure no matter how much you try to adjust the flavor. Don't worry! Just drink it and learn from that mistake.

The greens I most commonly use are bok choy, kale, mint, parsley, spinach, and Swiss chard. Spinach is a great choice for beginners as the flavor is mild and the green color often spectacular. Less often I use basil, beet greens, borage leaves and flowers, carrot tops, celery leaves, cilantro, fennel tops, purslane, radish tops, and romaine, but they are still excellent additions that can liven up a typical green smoothie. I have also experimented with regular salad mix when my "greens for green smoothies" container in the fridge runs low. Keep in mind that red leaves in salad mixes are generally bitter, and you may want to pick those out.

Don't use the same greens all the time; try different ones, and also rotate greens to respect the seasons. It is important to get a variety of nutrients and to avoid continually consuming the same plant-produced chemicals known as secondary metabolites (and sometimes called anti-nutrients). For example, Swiss chard and spinach contain oxalic acid, and if you use only these two greens, you may start to have problems. One issue with oxalic acid is that it binds with calcium, which decreases absorption of this important mineral. I can tell if I have been eating too much of the same greens because I start to not want smoothies and I feel a bit queasy midmorning. (See page 80 for more on the importance of variety.)

Making green smoothies is a snap if you wash the greens and have them ready to use ahead of time. Use just the leaves of greens with fibrous stalks like kale and chard (the stalks can be used finely sliced into salads or whole in soups and stir-fries). After washing the greens, air-dry them on dish towels and then put them in a large plastic container lined with a clean, dry towel before storing in the refrigerator. The towel absorbs excess moisture and stays hygienic for 5 to 7 days.

Try to buy organic greens, which are free of pesticides and herbicides and contain more nutrients than conventional greens. Farmer's markets are great places to find a variety of greens that aren't available in supermarkets. If you can only buy non-organic greens, please wash them very thoroughly. Even better, grow them yourself. Swiss chard is so easy to grow that even someone without a green thumb can do it! For those who have no land, large pots can be used very successfully in courtyards and on balconies.

What's the Big Deal About Greens?

Greens are rich in fiber, vitamins, minerals, antioxidants, pigments like chlorophyll (green) and carotenoids (yellow, orange, and red), and even essential fatty acids such as omega-3s. They are alkaline, low in calories, low on the glycemic index (see page 56 to find out why this is important), low in carbohydrates, and high in protein. Greens also aid digestion by stimulating digestive enzymes and help to normalize stomach acid.

According to Victoria Boutenko, pioneer of the modern-day green smoothie, greens are the primary foods that meet human nutritional needs most completely. Chimpanzees are the closest relatives of humans, with more than 99 percent of the same genes. They eat a diet made up of 50 percent fruit, 40 percent greens, and 10 percent pith, bark, and insects. Over 50 percent of the standard Western diet consists of cooked carbohydrates such as potatoes, bread, pasta, and rice. Approximately 35 percent is made up of fats, oils, and animal protein, and the remainder is fruits and vegetables, including greens. At best, the greens por-

Antioxidants

Greens are abundant in antioxidants, substances that protect us from illness, disease, and age-related conditions by defending cells against free radical damage. Free radicals are molecules or atoms with an unpaired electron in the outer shell; they are highly reactive and need to bond with something to stabilize their structure. Subsequently, free radicals create bonds that damage cell walls and internal cell structures such as DNA. Antioxidants prevent the free radicals damaging cells by making these bonds instead. Vitamins A, C, and E are examples of antioxidants, as are the color pigments found in plants, including chlorophyll and carotenoids. Find out more about antioxidants in "Superfoods in Green Smoothies" on page 88.

tion accounts for just a small percentage. The chronic diseases of humankind are not seen in wild chimps, so why not take a leaf out of their cookbook and see what their big secret is?

Greens for Salads and Smoothies

Greens are very hardy on a molecular level as their cell walls are made of cellulose. Nutrients are stored within the cells, and the walls need to be ruptured to release them. Breaking down the walls requires a significant amount of chewing, which we struggle to do as our jaw muscles have poor endurance and we are very impatient. We also need strong stomach acid, which many of us lack. Blending greens in a smoothie is the ideal way to get all the nutrients they contain, because a blender ruptures the cell membranes, releasing the nutrients very easily. I encourage you to eat greens whole in addition to using them in smoothies, but be sure to chew very well.

Although greens are incredibly abundant and diverse, many people are familiar only with lettuce and spinach. Incorporating a variety of leafy greens into your diet—in salads and smoothies—will ensure that the key nutrients of each are well distributed in your body.

Many types of greens are terrific in salads. They include arugula, baby beet greens, bok choy, butter lettuce, cabbage, cress, dandelion greens, endive, kale, lamb's lettuce, miner's lettuce, mizuna, mustard greens, oak leaf lettuce, radicchio, romaine, sorrel, spinach, Swiss chard, and tatsoi. Soft herbs such as basil, cilantro, mint, and parsley are also tasty in salads.

Greens that are great for smoothies are similar to salad greens; however, I recommend avoiding very bitter greens like radicchio and strong, hot-flavored ones like arugula, cress, and mustard greens as even sweet fruit won't overpower their flavors. Greens from the cruciferous family, including cabbage and kale, can be used in green smoothies. They contain antioxidants called indoles and cancer-fighting sulfur compounds known as isothiocyanates.

Extremely nutritious, microgreens and sprouts are commonly used in salads, but they are just as good in green smoothies. (See "Sprouts and Microgreens" on page 21 for more about growing microgreens and sprouts and using them in your smoothies.)

Many common backyard weeds such as dandelion, purslane, and chickweed are edible, too. Wild versions of cultivated foods such as wild fennel, endive, watercress, amaranth, and alfalfa also exist. Both types of greens are excellent sources of nutrients, frequently more nutritious than cultivated greens, and a great way to add variety to both salads and smoothies. If you do plan on using weeds or wild foods, be absolutely sure of what you are picking so you don't eat something poisonous. Get a good book or speak with an expert who can help identify the plants you hope to consume. Sergei Boutenko, son of Victoria, is a wild edibles expert and has produced videos and an iPhone app about wild greens. Visit www.sergeiboutenko.com for more information.

The same soft herbs you would use in salads can add amazing flavor to smoothies, and they have incredible nutritional properties with very high antioxidant values. See page 26 for more about using herbs in green smoothies.

Sprouts and Microgreens

Sprouts and microgreens are excellent in green smoothies and are super-nutritious. The flavors of microgreens and sprouts are surprisingly strong, so I suggest using a small amount in a smoothie in partnership with fully grown greens.

Sprouts and microgreens can be grown easily at home to supply nutritious greenery all year round. Microgreens are greens harvested as seedlings. Sprouts are germinated seeds with a very young root stem and usually pale leaves; lentil, alfalfa, and mung beans are common types of sprouts.

Sprouts

You can buy seed-sprouter kits and follow the instructions; however, I prefer to use the following method to sprout seeds myself. For small seeds, like alfalfa, start with about 2 tablespoons seeds. For larger seeds, like lentils (French puy or black beluga are best) or mung beans, start with ¼ to ½ cup seeds.

1. Cut a piece of fine netting like tulle or hosiery and fasten with a thick elastic band on top of a 1-quart glass jar.

2. Place the seeds in the jar, fasten the netting, and soak the seeds overnight in good-quality water.

3. In the morning, drain the liquid and rinse the seeds with cold water till the liquid is clear (you can use the soaking water to water other plants).

4. Let the jar sit and drain at a 45-degree angle on your dish rack. Rinse the seeds twice a day, three times if the weather is particularly warm. Avoid direct sunlight on the jars or the seeds will cook and go rancid. If the sprouts look or smell bad, throw them out and start again.

5. Sprouts of small seeds are ready in 5 to 6 days, when the tails are about 1 inch long. Rinse the hulls off in a colander, and pop the sprouts back into the jar to turn green in natural indirect light for about a day. Sprouts of large seeds are generally ready in 3 to 5 days when the tail is 1 to 2 times the length of the seed (the hulls of large seeds need not be rinsed. Spread the sprouts in a colander and leave to turn green in natural, indirect light for a day.

6. When the sprouts are ready, store them in the refrigerator in a container that can breathe a bit. Eat within a few days.

Alfalfa is Arabic for "father of all foods." It is one of Dr. Gillian McKeith's top-12 superfoods. She says alfalfa contains all the necessary nutrients for life, nourishes the blood, aids nutrient absorption, deodorizes the body, improves digestion, and is good for recovery after childbirth and for improving quality of breast milk.

Some sources call for sprouting to be in a dark place such as a cupboard to mimic the dark conditions of a seed germinating under the soil. I have found this not to be necessary, but I have experimented with covering my sprout jars with a tea towel or dish towel while they drain, and I believe my sprouts grow more quickly this way. I uncover them for the last day so they green up.

Lentils have the second highest protein content in a legume (after soy). They aid kidney and adrenal function due to good B vitamin content particularly, vitamin B1 and folate. They are also a good source of iron, phosphorus, and manganese and are a complete protein once sprouted.

Mung bean sprouts are well-known in Asian food dishes and are grown commercially under pressure and in the absence of light to create 2- to 3-inch tails with pale yellow leaves. When they are sprouted at home, they will still contain the green hull and have a short, stumpy tail. They are a good source of vitamin C, vitamin K, folate, manganese, and copper.

Before sprouting, check for small stones in seeds such as lentils, and check for mung beans that remain hard despite the sprouting process. You don't want to find one the hard way and chip a tooth!

Microgreens

Microgreens have larger stems than sprouts do, and clear leaf development with green leaves. They are harvested by cutting the leaves away from the root when they are 1 to 2 inches tall. Microgreens are grown in 1 to 3 weeks on soil or a soil substitute. Common microgreens are are wheatgrass, sunflower shoots, and cress. Basil, beet, and cilantro microgreens are very popular in restaurants for adding subtle flavor and garnish to dishes.

Items you'll need:
- Seeds, preferably untreated and nonirradiated
- Wide and shallow containers with drainage—these can be decorative ceramic dishes, seedling trays, or produce baskets with holes poked in the bottom
- Good-quality potting soil
- Cotton or paper towels
- Plastic or glass covers
- Water

To grow microgreens:
- Sprinkle seeds in a dense layer over potting soil in a container. (Soak any large seeds, like peas and sunflower seeds overnight before planting.)
- Cover the seeds with a light layer of the same soil mix, or place a damp cotton or paper towel over the seeds.
- Carefully water the seeds so as not to disturb them, like with a spray bottle. Cover the container with plastic or glass to create a greenhouse effect.
- Keep the seeds out of direct sunlight to avoid excessive heat. Microgreens can be grown outside in a protected spot or indoors, depending on available space and the temperature.
- Keep the seeds moist by watering 1 to 2 times daily. A spray bottle works well for watering gently.
- Keep the seeds covered until they germinate and start lifting the cotton or paper cover, or push through the soil coverage. Then remove the coverings and expose the germinated seeds to light and air. The greens will be ready to harvest in 7 to 21 days, depending on the

variety. To harvest, cut the baby plant stem off the root above the soil level.

- Ideally, use immediately after gently rinsing, or store in a zip-top bag or sealed container in the refrigerator for a day or two.

Growing microgreens and sprouts is great fun and makes the nutritious greenery for salad, garnishes, and green smoothies available to just about anyone. For those who are serious about growing microgreens and sprouts regularly, I recommend finding one or two books and websites to aid with troubleshooting and mastering a variety of greens. In her book *Microgreens: How to Grow Nature's Own Superfood*, microgreens expert Fionna Hill details the ideal conditions for growing amaranth, arugula, basil, beet, broccoli, cabbage, chives, clover, corn, cress, fennel, fenugreek, flaxseed, kale, mizuna, mustard, parsley, peas, radish, and wheatgrass.

And What About Herbs?

Tender, fragrant herbs are fabulous additions to green smoothies. Regular salad greens have either little or no taste or a bitterness that needs to be balanced by the sweetness and sometimes tartness of fruit. Herbs, however, add flavor as well as pack an amazing punch of nutrition and medicinal benefits.

There are hundreds of herb species and thousands of subspecies and varieties in gardens around the world, not to mention what is available in the wild. Whole books are devoted to herbs, so I will discuss the four most commonly available and most useful in green smoothies: basil, cilantro, parsley, and mint.

Because they contain volatile essential oils and antioxidant vitamins, flavonoids, and pigments, these four herbs have similar properties, including the ability to calm a stressed or anxious nervous system yet energize a system that requires stimulation. All four are digestive aids, are antibacterial and anti-inflammatory, and possess anti-cancer properties. They all contain varying degrees of vitamins C, A, and K as well as folic acid, iron, manganese, and calcium. Vitamin C is an antioxidant vitamin important for our immune system and soft tissue healing. Vitamin A is also an antioxidant vitamin necessary for our eyes, while vitamin K is vital for blood clotting and bone health. Folic acid is a B vitamin that has many roles to play, including the neurological development of a growing baby, the reproduction of DNA in our cells, and the stabilization of our mood. Iron is used in hemoglobin in our red blood cells. Manganese is necessary to facilitate enzyme reactions in the body, and calcium is vital for strong bones and for normal muscle contractions.

Basil

Derived from the Greek word meaning "royal," basil is the symbol of love in Italy. It is in the same plant family as mint and has similar medicinal properties to spearmint and peppermint in particular.

In addition to the attributes in common with cilantro, mint, and parsley, basil has an antispasmodic effect on the small intestine with its ability to relax the smooth muscle of its walls. Basil helps to increase circulation by dilating small blood vessels and is also considered an anti-worm agent.

The aroma of basil is good for memory and concentration, particularly in times of mental fatigue. Basil is particularly rich in vitamin K. It also contains zeathanthin, a carotenoid antioxidant that protects the eye.

Basil is warming and can have a clovelike taste. It goes well with the following green smoothie–friendly ingredients: cilantro, coconut milk, fig, ginger, lemon, lime, mint, and tomato.

GROWING AND STORING BASIL

Growing basil isn't hard, and being able to pluck a few leaves or a big handful is nothing short of wonderful. Home-grown basil tastes so much better than store-bought and is so much cheaper! I have found it's easier to grow basil successfully from seedlings than from seeds. Also, to get basil leaves for a good 4 to 5 months, the trick is to pick off the seed heads. Basil will keep trying to go to seed, but remove the seed heads every few days and you will get a bushier basil plant that seems to last forever.

Basil storage isn't as successful as storage of other herbs because the leaves bruise and turn black very easily. If you choose to grow basil yourself, just harvest leaves as you need them and use them immediately. If buying basil, store it unwashed in a dish towel–lined container in the refrigerator and wash as needed. Another option is to wash very gently, let air-dry, and store the same way. Use stored basil within 2 to 3 days.

Mint

In Greek mythology, Pluto was in love with the nymph Minthe. Pluto's jealous wife, Persephone, cast a spell on Minthe, turning her into a plant that she trampled upon. Unable to reverse the spell, Pluto gave his beloved a scent—the classic, dominant menthol aroma of peppermint—that became stronger the more it was stepped on.

Varieties of mint include spearmint, apple mint, pineapple mint, peppermint, and even chocolate mint. The benefits of mint aromatically and medicinally are almost identical to those of basil; however, stronger menthol oils, which produce the classic mint aroma, have a more powerful effect in calming an inflamed or spastic gut, and provide a cool, stimulating effect on the skin and to the taste. Menthol can be used as a mild analgesic on the skin and is frequently added to topical creams to ease muscular pain. Mint is commonly added to oral hygiene products because of its antibacterial and cleansing effects.

Mint contains organic compounds including perillyl alcohol, which has anti-tumor properties, and rosmarinic acid, which is particularly good as an anti-inflammatory agent for the airways. In addition to a broad spectrum of vitamins and minerals, mint also contains omega-3 oils, vitamin E, vitamin B2, potassium, and magnesium.

In green smoothies, mint goes well with basil, cilantro, citrus, cucumber, ginger, kiwi fruit, lemon, lime, melon, parsley, and tomato.

GROWING AND STORING MINT

Anyone who has grown mint knows it grows like a weed! Its root system spreads and new shoots continue to pop up; if left uncontained, it creeps. You can contain mint in pots, though it tends to get pot bound and is not as healthy as when grown in the ground. Either way it is worth planting because it is so very versatile as a culinary herb, adding wonderful taste and flavor to many dishes, including green smoothies. Mint can keep going year-round; it may die to the ground during winter in cooler climates, but it will come back in spring.

If you buy mint, keep the leaves on the stems and wash gently. Let the mint air-dry without going limp. Store in a dish towel–lined container in the refrigerator for 5 to 7 days.

Cilantro/Coriander Leaf

The leaves of this medicinal herb are known as cilantro in the United States and Latin America, and the seeds are known as coriander. In Asia, Australia, and the United Kingdom the leaves and seeds are both referred to as coriander. The leaves been used for thousands of years, as documented in ancient Egyptian and Sanskrit writings.

In addition to possessing the usual herbal properties (anti-bacterial, anti-anxiety, anti-cancer, anti-inflammatory, and a digestive aid), cilantro is considered a good herb for diabetics as it helps to regulate insulin activity. It also helps lower cholesterol by improving the digestion of fat.

Cilantro is rich in chlorophyll, making it a great chelator of heavy metals and toxins—meaning it attaches to the toxin to disarm it and remove it safely from the body.

Because cilantro has a very strong flavor, people usually either love it or hate it. If you are like me and you love it, then you'll eat this magnificent herb with gusto! Even if you are not a big fan, you can still receive the benefits by combining it with greens and other herbs, particularly mint or parsley. In addition to a substantial variety of vitamins and minerals, cilantro also contains the antioxidant flavonoid quercetin, which has antiviral, anti-inflammatory, and anti-allergy properties.

In green smoothies, cilantro goes well with avocado, basil, beet, coconut, cucumber, ginger, kiwi fruit, lemon, lime, mint, parsley, and pineapple.

GROWING AND STORING CILANTRO

One of the most challenging herbs to grow, cilantro is renowned for bolting, or going to seed, very quickly. In my experience, even the slow-bolting variety still bolts! The best results I found came from sowing coriander seeds kept in the pantry and typically used in cooking. My mother tried this with some seeds that were quite old. They grew and she had the best cilantro ever! In general, though, this is one herb I tend to let the experts grow, and when frequenting farmer's markets, I buy many bunches and have a lot of cilantro that week.

Because cilantro often has a lot of grit and sand when you buy it, wash it several times. Fill a sink and gently swish the leaves around to release the dirt. Repeat until the water stays clear. Gently shake off excess water or put it through a salad spinner, air-dry, and store in a dish towel–lined container in the refrigerator. How long the herb lasts depends on how fresh it was when stored. It may last a few days or more than a week. Bright, intact roots are a good sign.

Parsley

A member of the celery and carrot family, parsley was held in such high esteem by the ancient Greeks that they adorned athletic victors with it.

Parsley is very high in the green pigment chlorophyll, which is a detoxifier or chelator of heavy metals, and a deodorizer, masking the odor of other foods. Chewing parsley after eating a pungent dish such as one with garlic helps to freshen breath. Along with high levels of chlorophyll, parsley also has high amounts of antioxidant vitamins and flavonoids. The flavonoid luteolin has anti-cancer properties and is an important antioxidant for the blood. The volatile oil myristicin facilitates the function of glutathione, the most important antioxidant in the liver.

This herb is also rich in vitamin A and in carotene pigments such as zeathanthin, both necessary for eye health. High amounts of vitamin C and iron make parsley an excellent source of iron for vegetarians, because non-heme iron (which comes from plants) is harder for the body to absorb than heme iron (that found in animal foods), and vitamin C increases the uptake of iron in the body. High levels of vitamin K and folic acid mean parsley is excellent for cardiovascular heath.

Parsley is an excellent source of vitamins A, K, and C. It also contains all of the B vitamins in addition to a wide variety of minerals. Parsley is excellent for detoxification due to its very high antioxidant vitamins, flavonoids, and pigments.

In green smoothies, parsley goes well with: avocado, cabbage, cardamom, cilantro, citrus, cucumber, kale, kumquat, lemon, mint, and pomegranate.

GROWING AND STORING PARSLEY

Anyone who has grown flat-leaf, or Italian, parsley knows that after one successful crop, you will have it forever. When the plant goes to seed, it grows a massive flower head containing hundreds of seeds. If left to dry and drop naturally, the seeds will produce more plants all by themselves. In warmer climates, parsley tends to have two seasons a year, but if you plant crops about 2 to 3 months apart, you will have parsley all year.

Parsley is quite robust when it comes to washing and storage. You don't need to handle it as gently as you do basil, mint, or cilantro. You can store parsley on the stems, or pick off the leaves and tender stems from the woodier ones. Wash and shake off excess water or put the parsley through a salad spinner. Air-dry and store in a dish towel–lined container in the refrigerator. Freshly harvested parsley has lasted up to 2 weeks for me this way. If the parsley is going limp or turning yellow, throw it out.

To Juice or Blend?

Ask juice experts and smoothie experts this question and they will extol the virtues of their bias in a convincing fashion, enough that you begin to go down either pathway with confidence. However, is one method better than the other? The main pro-juice argument is that the absence of fiber provides easy assimilation of concentrated nutrients straight into the bloodstream with little digestion required. The other side of this debate is that the presence of fiber in smoothies is the unique selling point.

The late Dr. Ann Wigmore, a nutritional pioneer, advocated a diet that was 70 percent blended smoothies and 30 percent other living foods. She lived an extremely healthy and fit life, and reportedly had no gray hair. Best-selling author Steve Meyerowitz, "the sprout man" teaches that consuming fresh juices conserves the body's digestive energy, so more energy can be spent on healing. Interestingly, Ann Wigmore said the very same thing. They both speak of pre-digestion and the provision of a high level of nutrition from their preferred drink.

Juices do not contain fiber, so their nutrients are absorbed very quickly, high in the digestive tract. The job of the digestive system is to break down foods so they can be absorbed, but with juices there's nothing to break down. No chewing is needed and little or no digestive energy is required. Smoothies are essentially juices with blended fiber—and it is the presence of fiber in smoothies that proponents of the drinks point to as their main virtue.

There are two types of fiber in foods: insoluble and soluble. Insoluble fiber is the roughage that keeps a person from getting constipated and helps to control the pH (acid-alkaline balance) in the intestines. Both of these functions are extremely important when it comes to preventing bowel and colon cancers. Soluble fiber attaches itself to LDL cholesterol (low-density lipoproteins, considered the "bad" cholesterol), removing it from the body via the intestines. In addition, it helps to bulk up the stools and keep them soft. Soluble fiber also helps maintain blood sugar levels by prolonging stomach-emptying time; thus it's beneficial in maintaining energy and in helping regulate blood sugar disorders such as diabetes.

Neither type of fiber is absorbed by the body; after serving its purpose in the digestive tract, fiber is excreted in feces. Insoluble fiber—found in particularly high levels in green, leafy vegetables, for example—is broken down into smaller pieces, but it passes through the intestines essentially intact on a molecular level without being used for energy or nutrition. Soluble fiber, rich in foods such as flax and chia seeds, forms a gel in water and also passes through the digestive system without being absorbed.

Let's look at an orange consumed three ways: juiced, blended, and eaten. Orange juice requires no chewing and little or no energy beyond the stomach, and all of the sugars, vitamins, minerals, and antioxidants are available immediately and absorbed quickly into the bloodstream. A blended orange requires no chewing and minimal energy in the stomach and intestines, since the fiber has already been broken down into very small and functional pieces. The same nutrients as in the juice are absorbed more slowly, and the sugars are released more slowly into the bloodstream because of the presence of soluble fiber. By comparison, eating an orange requires breaking down all of the constituents into smaller pieces, starting with chewing, then churning in the stomach, and further liquefying in the intestines so the fiber is small enough to do its job and the nutrients and sugars are small enough to be absorbed.

I've observed that people tend to chew as few as 2 or 3 times and up to about 10 times, yet 20 to 50 chews per bite are recommended. Although such little chewing may save jaw energy, it's at the expense of the rest of the digestive system: chewing keeps the stomach and intestines from working so hard and stimulates the production of digestion enzymes further down the chain. Poor chewing can lead to incomplete digestion, which sacrifices the absorption of nutrients and can lead to an excess of bacterial growth in the gut. Most of us eat much too quickly, for reasons such as eating on the run, eating without thinking (like while in front of the TV), and lack of jaw muscle endurance. Try chewing everything 50 times! It's exhausting and time consuming. We would develop much stronger jaws—not a bad thing, but in reality we just don't chew enough and we are very unlikely to start doing it. So it's not surprising that we have an epidemic of nutritional deficiencies and digestive disorders, which could be blamed on poor chewing habits.

It is pretty clear that, from a digestive standpoint, juicing or blending is better than eating. A caveat: Swirl the juice or smoothie in the mouth to stimulate saliva before swallowing; otherwise digestion further down can still be compromised.

Both juicing and blending provide a predigested and readily available supply of nutrients; the difference is that the fiber in smoothies slows the absorption of nutrients and sugars. The advantage of juices over smoothies is that when major nutritional deficiencies are present or the constitution very weak, bypassing the intestines helps the body rest its digestive energies and heal. Also, some people don't tolerant fiber well as it irritates their intestines, so juices are a good choice for them.

If none of these conditions are present, then smoothies offer many advantages, principally fiber. Most people do not eat the recommended 25 to 30 grams of fiber daily. Some sources suggest we consume as much as 45 grams per day. The average daily consumption in the United States is 12 to 18 grams; in Australia it is approximately 20 grams, and in the United Kingdom 12 to 16 grams. Western countries, where the rates of high cholesterol, Type 2 diabetes, constipation, and colon cancers are high, all have recommendations to increase fiber in the diet for disease prevention and treatment.

Smoothies are filling, so they can be a meal. Smoothies are most often eaten for breakfast, and since this is a time when people are in a hurry, smoothies are a fabulous time-saver as well as an excellent source of nutrition to start the day. You can blend a smoothie and clean the blender in just minutes. Juicing is time consuming. A masticating juicer, which is slow but provides better-quality juice than a centrifugal juicer, can take up to 30 minutes to make juice—and then you have to clean the juicer! This is the bane of everyone who uses a juicer. Even if you have a fast centrifugal juicer, cleaning it still takes much more time than cleaning a blender. Many people start juicing but before long stash the juicer in the cupboard because it's a nuisance.

Smoothies produce little or no waste. Apart from peels from fruits like bananas and some tough stalks from greens, your compost pail won't fill up when you make a smoothie. The same cannot be said for juices because of the fiber, which is usually discarded.

Juices are not particularly filling. Have a juice for breakfast and you will be hungry in an hour. Commercially prepared juices made fresh from raw ingredients are usually consumed in addition to a meal or to quench thirst, adding unnecessary calories because they are high in sugars. They lack fiber, which slows stomach emptying and keeps sugars from getting into the bloodstream too quickly. Instead sugars rapidly enter the blood, providing a surge of energy followed by a drop later on. By comparison, consuming sweet foods and drinks containing fiber—in the form of smoothies—helps regulate blood sugar and aids in weight control.

Consuming greens in your smoothie supercharges this blood-sugar balancing effect by adding more fiber to the mixture than exists in whole fruit alone, and furthermore the high protein content of greens helps slow carbohydrate digestion. This means steadier blood sugar for longer, which makes you feel more satisfied between meals and less likely to overeat or snack. For more about carbs and their effect on blood sugar, see "Crazy About Carbs" on page 54.

The History of Blending

More than a century ago, "smoothie" described a man who was a charmer or sweet talker. The word has served as a brand name for pens, chocolate syrup, whiskey, lingerie, automotive paint additive, shoes, and soft drinks. It also refers to hairless nudists!

As we know it today, a smoothie is a thick drink that contains fruit blended with juice, milk, or yogurt. Although various people claim to have come up with the name for commercial purposes—most notably Stephen Kuhnau, founder of Smoothie King in the 1970s—the smoothie really dates back much further. The Indian *lassi*, a creamy blend of yogurt, fruits, and spices, could well be the world's first smoothie, originating around 1,000 BC. In the 1920s and 1930s, pureed fruit drinks based on recipes from Brazil were sold in health food stores on the U.S. West Coast. In the late 1920s, Orange Julius evolved from selling just orange juice to orange juice mixed with milk, sugar, and vanilla. An improvement on the mixers and liquefiers of the 1920s, the world's first blenders were released in the 1930s, most famously by Waring, which produced the "miracle mixer" in 1933 and the "Blendor" in 1937 and in the 1940s featured smoothie recipes in its cookbooks. The founder of Vitamix also released a machine, the Blender, in 1937.

Smoothies rose in popularity in the 1960s and mainly featured a combination of fruit, fruit juice, and ice. The 1970s saw the addition of frozen milk and yogurt, and in the 1980s adding supplements became commonplace. In the 1990s the smoothie and juice bar industry exploded, and today it's worth billions of dollars. Juice and smoothie franchises, including Smoothie King and Jamba Juice, abound.

In 2004, Victoria Boutenko introduced what is now known as the green smoothie. Having eaten 100 percent raw foods for a decade, Boutenko and her family report healing themselves of illnesses and diseases such as rheumatoid arthritis, diabetes, thyroid disease, morbid obesity, asthma, and allergies. However, they were not satisfied with their way of eating, and even though they were so much healthier than before, they knew something was missing. Boutenko's passion and talent for thorough research led her to conclude that the missing element in their diet was leafy greens. She researched the diet of chimpanzees, our closest genetic relatives, and compared it to typical diets of raw foodists and those eating a standard American diet. She discovered that the chimpanzee diet is approximately 50 percent fruit and 40 percent leafy greens. Although raw foodists ate a high percentage of fruit, they ate only around 10 percent greens. The standard American diet, she ascertained, was not only very low in fruit consumption but even lower in greens.

Boutenko calculated that her family would need to eat two bunches of greens and 4 to 5 pounds of fruit daily. While it was easy to eat a lot of fruit, they found it difficult to eat that many greens just in the form of salads. Once Boutenko learned that the tough cell walls of plants needed to be ruptured to release their abundant nutrients, she had a lightbulb moment: blend the greens with sweet fruit and water. The addition of the fruit offset the taste of the greens and also satisfied a person's nutritional need to consume both fruit and greens. The green smoothie was born! For more information about Victoria Boutenko, her books *Green for Life* and *Green Smoothie Revolution* are excellent resources.

Blending greens, however, was not a new concept. Many decades before Boutenko's moment of inspiration, Dr. Ann Wigmore, a pioneer of the raw food movement who developed seed cheeses and nut milks and also introduced the world to wheatgrass, was a big advocate of blended food. She called one of her blended raw soups that contained greens "energy soup." Although it has unlimited variations, the original recipe calls for rejuvelac, sprouts, leafy greens, avocado, seaweed, watermelon rind, carrot, and apple. Dr. Wigmore recommended eating 70 percent blended foods, believing this was the most efficient and easiest way to provide food that is both easy to digest and nourishing. She believed her blended recipes were a great way of maintaining good health, as well as helping sick people heal, as the digestive burden of regular eating was lifted, yet fiber and nutrients were delivered in abundance.

Historically, proponents of natural hygiene advocated blending over juicing, believing that juicing was a form of refinement. Removing the fiber made the food "less whole." Blended salad recipes often involved tomatoes, peppers, cucumber, zucchini, lettuce, celery, and fennel. A recipe may have included nutritional yeast, spices, or garlic and usually a fat such as cold-pressed oil or avocado. Whether a blended salad, Dr. Wigmore's energy soup, or a modern-day raw soup with greens, this type of blended food is not dissimilar to what has been called a savory green smoothie, which some people find appealing as an evening meal. (Try the recipes for savory green smoothies or soups on page 220.)

Just as the smoothie industry has grown exponentially, green smoothies have also risen rapidly in popularity. There is a plethora of books, websites, and blogs devoted to the humble green smoothie. In less than a decade after Victoria Boutenko's lightbulb moment, the green smoothie is no passing fad; it is here to stay and getting stronger by the day!

What About a Blender?

Any blender can be used to make green smoothies, but less expensive ones will break down sooner. Two popular, very effective, though expensive brands are Vitamix and Blendtec. Personally I use a Thermomix, a multipurpose kitchen appliance that blends, processes, cooks, steams, warms or melts at 98.6°F (37°C), weighs, crushes ice, mills grain, and more. Single-purpose food processors will not work for smoothies. For traveling, the Tribest Personal Blender is a great tool as it is small and portable and includes drinking cups.

To incorporate the fiber well, you must blend green smoothies longer than you would conventional smoothies, which contain just fruit and liquid. A heavy-duty blender such as a Thermomix, Blendtec, or Vitamix is required for breaking down vegetables like celery and high-fiber parts of fruits such as a pineapple core. These blenders can easily crush ice. Ice also keeps the temperature of the blended liquid from rising in the Vitamix, Blendtec, or less expensive blenders.

Vitamix and Blendtec customers report that without ice, smoothies blended for 1 minute are warm and for 2 minutes very warm. Furthermore, these blenders are marketed as capable of making steaming hot soup from the friction of the blades when blended between 3 to 9 minutes. A warm smoothie is unpleasant, and the heat may destroy nutrients and enzymes. I blend green smoothies for up to 2 minutes in my Thermomix, and they never come out warm. If a smoothie became warm from friction alone, the temperature light would activate, warning me.

Less expensive blenders can make the contents warm too, but lengthy blending also tends to heat the motor, sometimes producing an electrical burning smell. This will make you rest your blender to keep your smoothie from getting warm, but it is rather annoying!

Top Tips for Blending Green Smoothies

Thermomix is my number one for quality, power, functionality, and temperature control. It is, however, the most expensive.

For all other blenders, experiment with the settings and use of frozen ingredients to avoid a warm smoothie.

For less expensive blenders:

- Rest the blender if you detect a burning smell or the base feels warm.
- Chop the ingredients into small pieces before adding to the jug.
- Ensure there is enough liquid for the solids to move because a very thick smoothie puts stress on a less expensive blender.
- Try blending the greens and liquid first before adding the fruit.
- Minimize frozen ingredients because the blades and motor may not handle them. Ensure frozen ingredients are in small pieces.

No matter the type of blender, it's best to minimize the use of frozen ingredients to avoid really cold smoothies—to avoid unnecessary strain on your digestive system.

Frozen ingredients should be used with caution. Yes, freezing excess ingredients and buying frozen items out of season is convenient—and there is no doubt that adding a frozen banana to a smoothie is like adding a scoop of ice cream!

In both traditional Chinese and Ayurvedic medicine, the consumption of very cold foods and drinks is not recommended. They describe digestion as a warm event, which increases activity. The consumption of cold fare supposedly slows digestion and requires additional, unnecessary energy to heat up to body temperature—consuming food that is frozen rather than merely cold obviously worsens the problem. There are also suggestions that very cold ingredients may affect the absorption of nutrients such as vitamin B12.

I am not a fan of ice in drinks, and I really dislike cold water from the refrigerator. I also know that if I use frozen ingredients in a smoothie, then the smoothie can be quite cold (because the Thermomix does not warm with friction); my solution is to add warm water rather than drink a very cold smoothie. Using large amounts of ice or frozen fruit in other types of blenders will also result in very cold smoothies. In order to make a green smoothie that is not too hot but is instead perfectly cool, be sure to go easy on ice and frozen ingredients and to be aware of your blender's mixing abilities.

Raw Foods

A raw food diet is about eating plant-based foods that are uncooked. That is, raw fruits, raw greens and vegetables, nuts and seeds. Specifically, "raw" means no heat is applied above 118°F (48°C). Heating above this temperature destroys all enzymes, denatures around 50 percent of protein, and destroys many vitamins and some minerals. For the purposes of this book, green smoothies are raw by this definition unless otherwise noted.

The obvious advantage of raw food is that it is more nutritious. One of the main theories about its benefits is that enzymes are preserved and thus the body requires less of its own reserves to digest the food. This theory does have its critics, and I am not totally convinced of its validity. However, there are more benefits to a raw food diet than just the enzyme factor.

At the heart of the diet are organic, unprocessed, whole foods, which means that raw foodies avoid pesticides, herbicides, and other chemicals in their foods. Foods known to be allergenic or to cause food intolerances, such as wheat, gluten, dairy, and soy, are generally not eaten or eaten minimally.

- Raw foodies tend to drink filtered or spring water, avoiding chemicals in tap water.

- Cookware is not used, eliminating the potential consumption of toxins from surfaces like Teflon and aluminum.
- Raw foodies don't eat meat and dairy products (or eat them very minimally). The consumption of animal protein above 10 percent of the total diet has been clearly linked to the diseases of affluence such as breast and prostate cancers, diabetes, and cardiovascular diseases.
- Raw foodies tend to avoid plastics and to use glass instead for drinking and storage. They also don't heat food in microwave ovens, which is commonly done using plastic containers.
- Avoiding chemicals usually extends to using chemical-free personal care products, as well.

Raw foodies also tend to be a healthy body weight. Toxins are stored in body fat when the organs can't cope with metabolizing them. If many toxins are present, then more fat gets laid down, especially around the hips. Fat also acts as an endocrine gland, producing more estrogen than is needed, potentially leading to estrogen dominance. Considering that raw foodies have a low toxic load and usually low body fat, the risk of estrogen dominance is low. Estrogen dominance may cause hormone imbalance in men and women, and the greater the exposure to estrogen, the higher the risk of diseases such as breast and prostate cancer.

A minority of people following a raw food diet eat 100 percent raw food, and some of their testimonials about recoveries from illnesses and obesity are remarkable. Most eat what is referred to as a "high raw diet," which is what I do. This means the majority of the diet, around 80 percent, is raw. I was introduced to raw by my mother, who successfully lost weight in middle age and kept it off for the first time in her life. Naturally I was curious, read a lot, and could not ignore what seemed to be such a logical path nutritionally. At times I have been 100 percent raw and had striking outcomes such as balancing hormones and conquering candida. I am willing to admit that it is very difficult to sustain a 100 percent raw diet, especially if you're social or when the weather is cold and wet in winter. Also, I think most of us have an addiction to and fascination with cooked food on many levels. My husband is supportive, but many couples and families struggle when there is no unison with food choices in the home.

In 1930, Paul Koukachoff, a Swiss medical doctor, studied the effects of cooked food on the blood. He discovered that eating food that had been heated to a certain temperature increased white blood cells, a process he referred to as digestive leukocytosis. White blood cells are the key to the human immune system; they increase when they are fighting diseases or foreign material in the body. Dr. Koukachoff found that eating unheated, raw food did not increase the number of white blood cells the way cooked food did. He also ascertained that eating at least half of the meal raw meant that no response was initiated. That research led to the recommendation, still followed today by many raw foodists, to eat at least half of each meal raw. This can be done simply by consuming a raw salad of some sort with each meal.

It is quite easy to maintain a very satisfying high raw diet by having a large green smoothie for breakfast, a large green salad at lunchtime, and a half raw/half cooked dinner. A breakfast consisting of 2 cups (500 mL) of green smoothie should see you through to lunchtime with ease. Your lunchtime salad should be a good volume to be filling and can be bulked up with half an avocado, some olives, or a tablespoon of seeds such as sunflower or pumpkin, which will add important fats and protein. A dressing containing flax, chia, or walnut oil will add necessary omega-3 fatty acids.

Dr. Fred Bisci, who has a doctorate in nutritional science and is a thriving 100 percent raw foodist in his 80s, appreciates that a 100 percent raw diet is not for everyone. He has a great eating plan for people who consume both cooked and raw foods: eat the raw before the cooked, and also stay within your chosen parameters. For example, if you pick an 80 percent raw, unprocessed, gluten-free diet, then stick to it. If you try to eat a higher percentage of raw food but that diet doesn't mesh with your lifestyle, then you won't stay with it. Allowing yourself occasional treats of junk foods or gluten-based foods will not do you any favors, either. Choose parameters that are necessary for your health (for instance, gluten free if your body doesn't tolerate gluten), and then make other healthful choices that work for your lifestyle. It is better to be consistently 80 percent or even 50 percent raw than it is to constantly change your diet.

A green smoothie for breakfast is the key meal within my parameters that keeps me on track and remaining high raw. If I eat just fruit for breakfast, it's never enough, and I crave more food later in the morning—which is not practical in my job as a busy physiotherapist. A gluten-free cereal or even raw granola just doesn't agree with me. My energy is low and I still feel the need for something else in mid- to late morning. I know some people thrive on a grain-based breakfast, but I don't. Having a green smoothie every morning suits my time constraints, satisfies my hunger and gives me a feeling of fullness, and my husband feels the same way. According to him, his day is not right unless it starts with a green smoothie!

The Protein Myth

One of the questions that vegetarians and vegans regularly get from people who know far less than they do about nutrition is, where do you get your protein from? After waiting for their blood to stop boiling from being asked *again*, they smile and politely reply that they get it from their food.

Seriously though, there is little danger of protein deficiency if you eat a variety of nutrient-rich foods. There is no need to focus concern on protein consumption when the real importance is on eating a nutrient-rich diet overall, whether for vegetarians and vegans, or meat-eaters. If your diet is balanced and you are getting all your nutrients (whether from animal products or other sources), you will be healthy.

The World Health Organization states that we need only 10 percent of our calories from protein. Dr. T. Colin Campbell, professor emeritus of nutritional biochemistry at Cornell University and author of the amazing book *The China Study*, says that we actually need only 5 to 6 percent of our calories from protein, but recommends 10 percent to ensure we get the smaller percentage.

We need carbohydrates primarily for energy, fat for the brain and endocrine system, and protein for growth and repair. As adults, we do not grow as we did as children, and definitely not the way we did as babies. Mother's milk is the perfect food for an infant up to 6 months of age, and it derives around 6 percent of its calories from protein—only 6 percent at the most rapid period of growth in life! Mother's milk is mostly fat and much of it is lauric acid, which is similar to the extremely healthy fatty acids in coconut water.

Many fad diets are high in protein and low in carbohydrates, in the mistaken belief that excreting ketones in urine is a good thing. Aside from overtaxing the kidneys, a high-protein diet reportedly leads to problems such as kidney stones, osteoporosis, mood disorders, and bad body odor. A high-protein diet does tend to cause weight loss, primarily due to calorie deprivation and the fact that protein is more filling than carbohydrate-based food of the same volume.

It is important to eat protein at each meal if you wish to lose weight and keep your blood sugar levels even; however, this does not mean a slab of meat at each sitting. Protein-rich plant sources are very abundant and include green leaves as well as sprouts such as alfalfa and lentil, nuts and seeds like almonds and sesame, legumes like chickpeas, and seed grains such as quinoa, chia, and amaranth.

The idea that you have to combine different plant-based protein sources to make a complete protein—for example, combining beans and rice—was debunked in the 1970s. As long as you regularly consume a variety of protein sources, it is not necessary to consume all essential amino acids in one meal.

What are amino acids? They are the building blocks of protein. When you eat protein-containing foods, your digestive system breaks down the proteins into individual amino acids and then reassembles them into new proteins, such as enzymes needed by the body. There are 22 amino acids, 8 of which are essential, meaning you must eat them because the body can't manufacture them. Complete proteins, for instance, meat and eggs, contain all 8 essential amino acids. The problem is that most concentrated protein sources are cooked, and cooking destroys 50 percent of the available protein. Although the cooked protein may be complete, it is only half available once eaten. Protein in raw plant foods are 100 percent available after eaten, and some plants such as soy, quinoa, chia, and amaranth are also complete proteins.

A big misconception is that people wanting to put on muscle need to eat more protein, and some bodybuilders consume extraordinary quantities of lean chicken breast, egg whites, or protein powder shakes. Yes, protein is necessary for growth, but what builds muscle is weight-bearing exercise or resistance training—and fuel is needed to do this. Copious amounts of chicken will fuel your body, but it's a much harder fuel to process than carbohydrates. Exercise and complex carbohydrate intake is the best combination because carbs are an energy-efficient fuel.

Green smoothies that consist of 40 percent greens are a great source of protein. Greens are protein rich: just look at grazing animals like cattle and sheep, not to mention apes. How muscular are these animals, and they are vegan! Spinach derives 30 percent of its calories from protein compared with cheese at 26 percent, milk at 23 percent, and beef at 50 percent. But remember, cooking destroys protein by 50 percent, so 3.5 ounces (100 grams) of cooked beef is similar to around 2.8 ounces (80 grams) of raw spinach for available protein content. Popeye couldn't be wrong, could he?

Crazy About Carbs

Living in our society, you could easily believe as many do that carbohydrates are evil. God forbid we eat any carbs because we will all end up obese! The world *is* getting more obese, but are carbs to blame? We live in a world of dietary confusion. Should we eat low carb or high carb? Low fat or high fat? High or low protein ? Low GI or low GL? There is no mention yet of whether or not these diets are omnivorous, vegetarian, vegan, or raw, or how the role of exercise plays in and what the differences are between men, women, and children.

What makes our attitudes about carbohydrates even more confusing is that not all carbs are the same. When low-carb diets refer to carbs, they usually mean starchy carbs and sugar. Some of these diets exclude fruit, and some exclude grains.

So what on earth are carbohydrates? Technically, they are saccharides, meaning they contain carbon, hydrogen, and oxygen in their molecular structure. Carbohydrates include a huge variety of structures from simple to complex. At the simple end are sweet-tasting monosaccharides, such as glucose and fructose, and disaccharides, consisting of two molecules joined together—for example, glucose plus fructose equals sucrose, otherwise known as table sugar. Then there are the non-sweet oligosaccharides, which consist of medium chains of sugar molecules in such foods as beans, and polysaccharides, which are long strings of monosaccharides or disaccharides, such as starch, glycogen, and cellulose. All carbohydrates must be broken down into a mono form to be utilized by the body as fuel.

Glucose is the carbohydrate found in the bloodstream, providing an immediate source of energy to cells and tissues. Fructose is metabolized by the liver, which stores it as glycogen and then releases it as needed into the bloodstream in the form of glucose. Excess fructose is metabolized into fat, which can be stored in the liver, potentially creating a fatty liver and sending fats into the blood as triglycerides—not ideal for good health.

In nature, sweet foods such as cane sugar, or sucrose, have a balance of glucose and fructose to provide both immediate and slowly released energy. Complex carbohydrates like the starches in root vegetables and processed grains contain many linked glucose molecules. They take longer than sweets to break down but provide a high level of glucose-based fuel. Very complex carbs like fiber are not broken down into absorbable molecules and exit the body via the bowel, serving very important roles along the way (see page 00). Starches found in nature, such as in root vegetables, also contain fiber; when eaten as whole foods, they slow down the absorption of glucose into the bloodstream.

The main problem with carbohydrates is refining and processing. Nature designed carbohydrates in forms that work for the body. Sweet foods like fruits contain a balance of simple sugars, and grains and vegetables a balance of starch and fiber. When you eat processed breakfast cereals that have had the bran, germ,

Glycemic Rankings

The glycemic index ranks carbohydrate-containing foods on a scale of 0 to 100 based on how much they raise blood sugar levels after they're eaten. Foods with a high GI ranking (above 70) are quickly digested and absorbed, causing blood sugar levels to fluctuate markedly. Low-GI foods (less than 55) are digested and absorbed slowly, producing gradual increases in blood sugar. The GI was developed in 1981 by David Jenkins, professor of nutrition at the University of Toronto, and has been an integral part of diabetes management and weight loss diets ever since. However, a newer and more valuable measure of the effect of carbohydrates on the body is glycemic load, developed in 1997 by Walter Willet, epidemiologist and nutritionist of the Harvard School of Public Health. It takes into account the glycemic index of a food as well as the amount being eaten. The GI rating is the same whether you eat 10g or 1kg so there are limitations to the concept of a low GI diet, because eating low GI can still mean eating too many calories. Subsequently, some foods like watermelon have a high GI and a low GL. Watermelon has a GI of 76 and has 5g of carbohydrate per 100g. Hence a serving of 100g of watermelon has a GL of 3.8 (5 x 76/100 = 3.8), which means a low GL. Eating 1kg of watermelon (as is required for GI testing), would give you GL of 38, which is high.

GL levels and recommended daily allowances (RDA) are not yet standardized, varying from one expert to another. Patrick Holford from the Institute of Optimum Nutrition, rates low GL as 10 or less, medium as 11 to 14, and high as 15 or more. Other resources such as mendosa.com and nutritiondata.com refer to low as 10 or less, medium as 11 to 19, and high as 20 or more. The RDA for the Holford diet is 40 to 45, nutritiondata.com suggests 100, and the glycemic load diet by Rob Thompson suggests under 500 (equivalent number is 50). All of these sources rely on the extensive database of GI and GL compiled by Professor Jennie Brand-Miller and colleagues at the University of Sydney, Australia.

The presence of protein and fiber affect GI and GL levels. Both slow the absorption of sugars from the gut into the bloodstream. Thus, the more a food is processed and broken down before it is consumed, the greater the likelihood of higher GL. Cooking carbohydrates also causes more rapid release of sugars, particularly if the carbs are cooked long or at high temperatures. Eating raw, unprocessed foods is ideal for minimizing GL.

fiber, essential fats, and vitamins removed, what you are left with is mostly starchy carbohydrate, dosing you with a rapid supply of glucose. Consuming soft drinks made from high fructose corn syrup overburdens the liver with fructose. However, when you eat whole fruits, vegetables, and grains, you get a balance of nutrients that the body is designed to cope with—provided, of course, that you are not fructose or gluten intolerant.

Many people are intent on reducing or even eliminating carbs. Strictly speaking, no carbs would mean no sugar, no grains, no legumes, no fruits, and no vegetables. A carb-free diet would mean eating just fat and protein in nuts, meat, dairy, and eggs. Such a diet would be extremely difficult and fraught with danger in the form of nutrient deficiencies. For anyone concerned about carbohydrate intake, particularly if the intention is to avoid a high-fat and high-protein diet, then looking at the glycemic index (GI) or, even better, the glycemic load (GL) is the way to go.

When glucose hits the bloodstream, a number of things can happen. Ideally, a steady flow of glucose is available as fuel for cells, with some left over to store as glycogen in the liver and muscles. Glucose enters the cells facilitated by the hormone insulin, which is produced by the pancreas. Insulin is responsible for keeping blood glucose down. If the blood glucose level decreases in the absence of a food supply, then glycogen stores are activated by the hormone glucagon to create new glucose molecules, resupplying the blood.

When a steady stream of glucose enters the blood, then there is only a small need for insulin to take it where it needs to go. However, if there's a flood of glucose to the blood, then a lot of insulin is required to lower it. Excess glucose is converted to fat, which the body stores, resulting in weight gain.

If the body can't make enough insulin or cells have become insulin resistant (due to prolonged high exposure to high insulin), then blood sugar levels stay high. High blood sugar is toxic to the body in many ways. It feeds infections, promotes inflammation, and can damage arteries, the brain, the kidneys, and the eyes. These complications are typical of end-stage, poorly managed diabetes.

If not enough carbohydrates are in the diet to supply glucose and the glycogen stores are depleted, then fat is used as a fuel source. A by-product of creating new glucose molecules is the production of ketones. The kidneys use minerals such as calcium and potassium to help excrete ketones from the body via the urine. Over a long period this may lead to mineral deficiencies, potentially affecting bone density, cardiac health, and muscle function.

Thus, if blood sugar is too high, the excess glucose is stored as fat. If it's too low, the result can be fatigue and the perceived need to reach for sugary, high-glycemic snacks and stimulants like caffeinated drinks.

Calories in our food come primarily from fats and carbohydrates. It's difficult to eat more than 20 percent of calories as protein considering that protein-based foods also contain carbohydrates (grains and legumes) or fats (meat, cheese, and nuts). It's most efficient for the body to acquire calories from carbohydrates, but aim for low-glycemic carbohydrates, specifically those with a low glycemic load. Such carbohydrates are generally more nutritious as they are more likely to be whole or minimally processed foods. They're also an ideal energy source when training, exercising, or taking part in sports. Eating complex carbs derived from whole foods rather than simple sugary or starchy carbs, results in high energy, a great mood, excellent elimination (because the diet is high in fiber), good muscle tone, and quick recovery after working out.

Essentially, the human body is designed to digest whole foods, not fractionated (broken down into components) foods: foods that contains fats, proteins, and carbohydrates intact, bound together with vitamins, minerals, and antioxidants. Green smoothies are an excellent way to receive all of these vital nutrients in addition to a "healthy" dose of carbohydrates.

So Why Are Green Smoothies Good for Blood Sugar?

Green smoothies are a good source of carbohydrates and excellent for blood sugar levels because they:
- Contain fiber
- Are raw (uncooked)
- Contain protein from greens
- Can be easily made with a low glycemic load (except when using more than one large banana per person or with dates or honey as a sweetener)

Should Fats Go in a Green Smoothie?

Fat is part of every cell wall in the body. It insulates our internal organs and nerve fibers. It is used to make hormones. Our brain is 60 percent fat. Fat is required to assist absorption of minerals and the fat-soluble vitamins A, E, and K. It is an energy source when blood sugar supplies are depleted. Fat is satisfying when eaten as part of a meal as it is high in calories, and it helps food taste better.

Using fats in green smoothies and in the diet generally requires a clear understanding of which fats should and shouldn't be used. There is a lot of talk in the media and in the field of nutrition about good and bad fats, and not all the information is the same, which makes the issue confusing. Fats, butters, and oils all contain fatty acids in their structure; they simply have different names according to whether they are hard, soft, or liquid at room temperature.

What Are the Different Kinds of Fats?

A fat molecule, or "fatty acid" is a group of connected carbon, oxygen, and hydrogen atoms. A fat can be classified according to how long its molecule is and also how "saturated" it is. A medium-chain fat has 6 to 12 carbon atoms at the center of the chain; a long-chain fat has more than 12. The joins or "bonds" between the carbon and hydrogen atoms can be single or double. When the bonds are single, the fat is considered to be saturated, and when the bonds are double, unsaturated.

Saturated medium-chain fats that are green-smoothie friendly come from coconut and palm kernels. Animal fats such as butter, cream, lard, and tallow are saturated long-chain fats. Monounsaturated fats are long chains with one double bond, which are the omega-9 fats such as those in olive and canola oils. Omega-3 and -6 oils are long-chain, polyunsaturated fats, meaning they have more than one double bond.

The omega-3 fat alpha-linolenic acid (ALA) and the omega-6 fat linoleic acid (LA) are considered "essential fatty acids" because the body cannot synthesize them—they must be supplied by the diet. They are important for the brain, skin, joints, and the cardiovascular system. Green smoothie–friendly sources of both of these essential fats are from the oils of flax seeds, chia seeds, hemp seeds, pumpkinseeds, sunflower seeds, walnuts, and some leafy greens. The ratio of omega-3 to omega-6 oils is considered very important. Most people generally consume too much omega-6. The ideal ratio of omega-6 to omega-3 is 3 to 1. Higher ratios are reported to encourage inflammation and the adverse thickening of blood.

Saturated fats are hard or soft, and their structure is very stable. The more unsaturated a fat is, the more unstable its structure. Polyunsaturated oils are liquid and go rancid more easily than saturated fats like coconut. For this reason, the food technology industry developed the process of hydrogenation, which creates a partially saturated fat like margarine that is no longer liquid and has a long shelf life. This process runs the risk of producing trans fats, which have an altered molecular structure. Similarly, fats may be interesterified to reduce rancidity and alter the melting point. A triglyceride is three fatty acids joined together, and interesterification changes which three are joined.

Trans fats and interesterified fats (IFs) do not exist in nature and are not forms of fat that are useful to the body. According to nutritionist Cyndi O' Meara, in her report on the making of margarine, trans fats and IFs have been linked to increases in

---

The Skinny on Fats

Fats that should be avoided (bad fats)

- Hydrogenated fats, trans fats, interesterified fats (IFs)—Found in margarines and other fake butter products and shortening; described as "vegetable fat" in ingredient lists; frequently used in the commercial baking industry
- Highly processed vegetable oils such as canola, sunflower, safflower, corn, cottonseed, and soy—Processed with chemicals and frequently genetically modified

Fats that should be encouraged (good fats)

- Saturated fat from coconut
- Oils rich in both omega-3 and -6 such as chia seed, hemp seed, flax seed, pumpkinseed, and walnut oils; micro-algae; and the leafy green purslane
- Oils from fish and krill (if not eating a vegetarian or vegan diet)

Fats that should be used in moderation

- Unsaturated oils from olives, avocados, nuts, grains, and seeds other than those listed above
- Animal-based saturated fats from meat, butter, cream, and eggs
- Cold-pressed, certified-organic sunflower oil

---

cancer, diabetes, and obesity, and an increased chance of heart disease. IFs and trans fats adversely affect cholesterol levels, destroy essential fatty acids, and circulate in the blood as solids. These unnatural fats wreak havoc on our body.

Long-chain unsaturated fats such as those in seed and grain oils and long-chain saturated fats from animals are digested using enzymes from the pancreas and bile from the gall bladder. They are broken down to be absorbed, and if not immediately utilized will be re-formed into triglycerides as a form of fat storage in the blood or tissues of the body. Medium-chain saturated fats such as coconut are short enough to be directly absorbed and used as an efficient source of energy. Dietary sources of cholesterol only come from the saturated fats of animals, so the tendency to lump coconut in the same category as animal fat is flawed. Coconut is an extremely healthy fat that is cholesterol free, and because it is metabolized quickly by the body due to its shorter chain length, it is not fattening!

How Do Fats Affect Digestion?

If you choose to follow the rules of food combining, which theoretically makes digestion easier, then you don't eat fat with sugar, which makes adding fat to a green smoothie "against the rules." The classic recommendations with food combining are no acid foods or protein with starchy carbohydrates, and no fruit with anything else (except greens). The theory is that these foods combined may ferment in your stomach causing gas or abdominal discomfort. There are many other food-combining rules, which if followed could mean a very strict diet of mostly mono foods, eating one type of food at a time, such as only watermelon for breakfast. Personally, I believe that you can combine foods and that fats are fine in green smoothies. To explain why, let's look at what happens in your body when you eat.

Let's start at the beginning: the main constituents of food are fats, proteins, and carbohydrates, which are broken down through various mechanisms in the body. By chewing the food, your teeth break it down mechanically into smaller pieces. Amylase in the saliva begins to break down carbohydrates; salivary lipase starts digesting fats.

A healthy stomach is a highly acidic environment, ideal for protein digestion. The stomach itself secretes pepsinogen, which is activated by stomach acid to form pepsin, the necessary enzyme to start protein digestion. The churning action of the stomach moves the food around, which mechanically breaks it down a bit further.

Next, food moves to the small intestine where bile, which is produced by the liver from cholesterol and stored in the gall bladder, is dumped in to help break down fats. The effect is like soap suds on greasy dishes. Bicarbonate ions are released to neutralize the acidic stomach juices, making it more alkaline. The pancreas also secretes enzymes such as lipase into the small intestine to break down fats, trypsin to break down proteins, and amylase to break down carbohydrates. Further down in the small intestine and in the large intestine are beneficial bacteria and additional enzymes to break food down to small molecules that are used as building blocks to keep the body operating properly.

The arrival of food stimulates the secretion of digestive enzymes—as does the smell and thought of food. The mouth salivates, the stomach growls, and the pancreas is stimulated. The pancreas is responsible for secreting enzymes to digest protein, carbs, and fat. The thought of any food type will stimulate digestive enzymes, not just one type of enzyme for one type of food, so the way you think about food will affect the way your body processes it. There are a variety of things to consider when we talk about food digestion. A few interesting ideas are:

- The body prepares itself to digest all three major components of food at the same time, so it seems that our digestive system is well designed and equipped to deal with food combinations. For example, if you don't chew food properly, you don't start fat and carbohydrate digestion in the mouth properly.
- If you have low stomach acid, then the stimulation of pepsin is poor and you struggle to start protein digestion.
- If you think of food all the time, overeat, or eat foods devoid of active enzymes (that is, processed and cooked foods), you may deplete your pancreatic enzyme ability. This will affect digestion of all three groups.
- If your diet is too high in fats, particularly saturated animal fats and cooked fats, your liver will struggle to keep producing enough bile to store in the gall bladder for use in helping to digest fats. Hydrogenated and interesterified fats can adversely affect bile production. Conversely, the medium-chain saturated fat from coconut requires no bile at all.
- If you are low in beneficial bacteria, then bad bacteria proliferate, interfering with nutrient absorption and producing gas and bloating.

So if you eat without thinking about what you're doing (say, in front of the TV), neglect to chew food completely or swirl liquid in your mouth, have hypochloridia (low stomach acid), eat too many bad fats, don't supplement with probiotics or eat fermented foods, and consume no or very little raw food, then your digestive system is going to be very, very stressed.

Though I still believe it is beneficial to combine foods, I see the wisdom in the thinking that recommends against it. For instance, if your digestive system is stressed enzymatically, then it makes sense that eating one type of food at a time will be more comfortable. There is also the point that whole foods are not just protein or just carbohydrates, but rather they are combinations. Meat consists of fat and protein. Fruits are mostly carbohydrates, though they have small amounts of protein and fat. Leafy greens contain carbs and protein, and some contain essential fatty acids that we need desperately, such as omega-3 in mint and purslane. Beans and nuts are combinations of protein and fat.

So, if you choose to combine foods, here is the action plan that should work if you respect the design of your body:

- Think consciously about your food prior to and during eating, and be happy and calm when eating.
- Chew well, or if drinking, swirl the liquid in your mouth.
- Improve the level of stomach acid by eating more greens, drinking green smoothies, or drinking 1 tablespoon of apple cider vinegar or lemon juice in water prior to a meal.
- Make at least 50 percent of every meal raw, uncooked, plant-based foods.
- Use supplemental probiotics and/or fermented foods.
- Avoid interesterified and hydrogenated fats in margarines and processed baked items. Also avoid heating fats beyond their smoke point and re-heating fats. If not vegetarian, use animal fats in moderation.

• Don't overeat. The size of your two fists together is supposed to be the size of your stomach and the maximum amount you should eat in one go, three times a day.

I must add that food allergies and intolerances are a different story. Back when I didn't realize I had to cut out gluten and dairy, following food-combining principles worked for me—but now that I don't consume any gluten, dairy, or coffee and minimal sugar (my food intolerances), I can combine any foods and be fine. I can eat protein, carbohydrates, and fruit after or with meals. It won't matter whether you combine or don't combine foods if you eat an allergenic food or a food your body can't tolerate. Your body will be upset until you remove the offending food.

Now, back to the question of fats in your smoothie...go for it! Fat aids the absorption of fat-soluble vitamins such as A, E, and K, as well as in the absorption of minerals. These nutrients are rich in greens, so put a little fat in your green smoothie to boost nutrient absorption. Try coconut flesh, coconut oil, ground flax seeds, chia seeds, raw nuts, hemp seeds, tahini, avocado, nut milk, nut butters, or flax oil. You don't need much, no more than a tablespoon of concentrated fat per serving.

Can Green Smoothies Help with Weight Loss?

How to achieve and maintain a healthy body weight is not only a very popular health topic, but it is also fraught with emotion. Search the Internet for "weight loss" or visit a bookstore and the possibilities are endless, though the outcomes not necessarily successful. Sadness, denial, frustration, or anger may result from the inability to lose weight. Why can some people lose weight and not others? Why do some lose weight at the start, yet can't continue and don't succeed in the long run? Is it discipline, diet type, or body type?

For some, being disciplined to eat less and exercise more just works. For others, it doesn't. Some can't exercise because of illness or injury, which undoes the concept of "energy in, energy out." Most diet plans work initially, but not over the long term. Compliance issues aside, the main reason for initial weight loss with any regime is calorie restriction. It doesn't matter whether you eat a highly nutritious plant-based diet, a high-protein diet, a red-foods-only diet, or just muffins; if you give your body fewer calories than it needs, you will use up your glycogen stores and begin to break down your stores of fats to use as fuel.

The problem with calorie restriction is that the body has the ability to adjust and reduce its rate of metabolism as it recognizes it is being starved. Ongoing calorie restriction won't see ongoing weight loss; instead, a plateau will be reached. Some diet programs are getting wise to this by including lower-calorie and higher-calorie phases to try and combat this effect.

To understand how green smoothies can aid weight loss, let's look at different types of diets to see where long-term compliance and success go wrong.

High-Protein/Low-Carb Diet

This diet can be very high in fat, often animal fat. On this regime, you can't avoid fat, as high-protein foods generally are high in fat—for example, meat, dairy (especially cheese), nuts, and eggs. According to Dr. T. Colin Campbell in *The China Study*, a diet plentiful in animal protein is associated with all the typical diseases of the Western world, namely breast and prostate cancers, heart disease, diabetes, kidney stones, and osteoporosis. Burning fat as your primary fuel source results in the production of glucose from fat; ketones are a damaging by-product of this process. This type of diet is not a healthy choice for the body in the long term.

High-Carb/Low-Fat Diet

A camp within the raw food community promotes this way of eating, often referred as the 80/10/10 diet because 80 percent of the calories come from carbs, 10 percent from fat, and 10 percent from protein. That's a very limited amount of fat, and just a small handful of nuts, half a small avocado, or 1 tablespoon of oil fills the quota. Proponents claim this type of raw food diet is best for healing illness and for high-level exercise training, as the main fuel source consists of sugars from fruit, which are very easy to metabolize. A lot of fruit must be consumed in order to get enough calories. A version of this diet is 30BAD, which means 30 bananas a day! Some people love that much fruit, but the diet has strong critics.

One danger is weight loss and lethargy if not enough fruit is consumed. Another risk is a deficiency of essential fatty acids. The body needs some saturated fat and essential fats such as omega-3s and omega-6s. Fats make up cell walls, and they make hormones, including insulin, testosterone, estrogen, and progesterone. Without the right oils in your diet you may have issues not just with hormones but also with skin, joints, brain, and eyes. Essential fatty acid deficiency can lead to blindness, mental health disorders, and birth defects. Although the body does not have a high-protein requirement, it must get enough protein calories to avoid amino acid deficiencies. It must be said, however, that neither amino acid deficiency nor essential fatty acid deficiency is unique to this style of diet. Such issues can be common in diets with poor variety and consumption of fat sources that largely exclude essential fatty acids.

Low-GI Diet

As discussed in the chapter "Crazy About Carbs" (page 54), the glycemic index (GI) measures how much different carbohydrate-containing foods raise blood sugar levels after they're eaten. For many people, low-GI diets are successful for weight loss and controlling blood sugar. Moreover, eating a low-GI diet is considered easier as a long-term diet strategy for health compared with diets that have extremes of food proportions such as high carb or high protein. A drawback of the low-GI plan is that it does not necessarily take into account portion size and whether a low-GI food is actually healthy. Just as a vegan could live unhealthily on jam sandwiches, someone could live on fried meatballs and theoretically eat a low-GI diet. Of course, these are extreme examples, but a low-GI diet can still be high in fat and protein and present the same risks as a high-protein/low-carb diet.

Diets with Three or Four Phases

The Atkins plan now has four phases. The South Beach and Fat Flush Diets have three. All of these diets are designed with initial significant calorie and carbohydrate restrictions, followed by less strict maintenance phases. The Curves Diet Plan has three phases that involve initially reducing calories to lose weight, then increasing calories to keep the body's metabolism from slowing. Reverting back to earlier phases may be necessary to control unwanted weight gain and can potentially be done numerous times. None of these diets is particularly friendly to vegetarians, vegans, or people with food intolerances and the switching between phases can be very challenging to incorporate into work, social, and family life.

Raw Food Diet

A raw food diet calls for eating uncooked plant-based foods: raw fruits, raw greens and other uncooked vegetables, and unprocessed nuts and seeds. Specifically, "raw" means no heat above 118°F (48°C). Someone who is termed a "raw foodie" might eat either a high raw diet or a 100 percent raw diet (see page 46). Well-known raw food authorities such as Shazzie, Jingee Talifero, Alissa Cohen, and Angela Stokes all have remarkable stories of weight loss and health gain on a raw food diet.

What is distinctive about a raw food diet is not only the successful weight loss stories, but the testimonials about curing illness and disease, such as reversing diabetes, asthma, and arthritic symptoms. We don't usually hear such things about other diets, as the focus is more on losing weight than regaining health. Unfortunately, there seems to be just as much variation and opinion in raw food diet styles as there is in mainstream dieting—for example, high carb/low fat versus high fat/low carb, juice fasting, water fasting, green smoothies, superfoods versus no superfoods, and raw cacao versus no raw cacao. The answer is not as easy as "just eat raw food."

Why do people tend to lose weight so easily on a raw food diet, though? One of the many theories is that it is relatively low calorie. Those not concerned about staying low fat can actually eat a lot of fat and still lose weight and maintain quite easily. A raw food diet is generally very nutritious—and it's easier not to overeat when eating nutritiously. It's not hard to overeat cookies or chips, yet has anyone overeaten a green salad? A symptom of eating empty calories like processed, sugary products is the tendency to keep eating as the body craves nutrition but doesn't get it. A raw food diet may help with portion control if you have a penchant to overeat.

People eating raw foods sometimes describe going through a detox or healing crisis at the start of the diet or along the way. This may have to do with the release of stored toxins in the body. Toxins are stored in fat in the hips and abdomen and also the liver. As the body goes through detoxification with nutrient- and enzyme-rich foods, toxins are eliminated and the need to store extra fat is reduced. Because raw foodies tend to live a life that has a low toxic load, again there is less need for fat in which to hide toxins. This may also be a reason for the success of long-term weight loss associated with eating raw foods.

Looking at the issue of weight loss and weight gain scientifically, what is it we know for sure?

There is little doubt that control of blood sugar is paramount, and this concept underpins most diets. The more glucose that floods the blood, the higher the risk of storage as fat, because there is more glucose than is needed for fuel and for glycogen stores.

The body needs sufficient calories for fuel without side effects.

- Too much carbohydrate in the form of fructose can lead to the production of blood triglycerides and a fatty liver.
- Too much glucose in the blood raises insulin and can lead to fat storage, or the inability to produce enough insulin means high blood glucose, which is toxic.
- A high-fat/low-carb diet leads to high levels of ketones, which must be excreted, taking precious minerals with them.

The tendency to overeat can be stopped by:
- Nutrient-dense foods
- Fiber-dense foods
- A filling combination of protein and carbohydrates

Factors that influence steady blood sugar are:
- Fiber-dense foods, particularly those containing soluble fiber
- A combination of protein and carbohydrates
- Carbohydrates with a low glycemic load (GL)
- The minerals chromium, magnesium, and zinc
- The spice cinnamon
- The herb cilantro
- Vitamin C
- Avoiding stimulants such as stress and caffeine

The addition of green smoothies to non-raw food and raw food diets frequently results in better weight control, and it's easy to see why—green smoothies tick all the boxes for blood sugar control and a feeling of fullness. Green smoothies:
- contain fiber.
- are (usually) low GL.
- contain protein and carbohydrates.
- are highly nutritious.
- supply good-quality fuel for cells without side effects.
- are alkaline and thus calming (non-stressful) to the body.
- are often rich in vitamin C.
- are made from organic and wild food sources, meaning they are more likely to supply trace minerals that are low or absent in conventional produce.

Hello, Sweetie!

To say someone has a sweet tooth is a bit odd, considering that teeth are the only part of the mouth without taste buds. Saying you have a "sweet tongue" or "sweet roof of your mouth" doesn't sound too enticing, does it? The term "sweet tooth" originates from "toothsome," meaning pleasing to the taste. Sweetness is one of the five basic tastes along with bitter, salty, sour, and umami (savoriness). The pleasure we get in eating and drinking is very much tied to the balance of these tastes on our tongue, and "pleasure" indeed is the word most associated with sweetness.

To make green smoothies delicious, you have to balance any bitterness and sourness with sweetness. Make the smoothie with only whole lemons and parsley, or just greens and water, and you will struggle to drink it. Green smoothies need some sweetness to make them palatable enough to drink over the long term and in large enough quantities—at least 16 to 32 ounces, or 2 to 4 cups (500 mL to 1 liter), daily. Ideally, fruit will supply the sweetness, but not all fruit is sweet enough. If you use berries, tart apples, whole oranges (the white pithy parts are nutritious but bitter), pears that aren't fully ripe, or non-sweet fruits like cucumber, your green smoothie will taste primarily of the green you used, which might be a bitter flavor depending on the quantity of green. You could say a green smoothie is bittersweet, that is, a balance of pleasure and pain. Your green smoothie will be painful if you don't inject the right amount of pleasure, or sweetness!

What if the fruit isn't sweet enough? There are several ways to solve that problem. To put the various options into perspective, let's start by talking about plain old sugar. When most people think of sugar, they usually think of table sugar, or sucrose, which is 50 percent glucose and 50 percent fructose. However, "sugar" is really a general term for simple carbohydrates that are sweet, can be processed into crystals or syrups from a variety of plants (sugar cane, sugar beets, and corn starch), and exist naturally in many foods, such as fruits, vegetables, and dairy products.

An equal or lower glucose to fructose ratio suits our bodies to maintain energy. Glucose raises blood sugar quickly and gives us immediate energy; fructose releases energy more slowly as it has to be broken down by the liver. Sugars that contain a higher proportion of fructose and should be avoided include honey, fruit juice concentrates, dried fruits, and agave nectar (a very high-fructose, runny syrup made from the agave plant and a "sugar-free" alternative popular among vegans and in the raw food world). Although they are natural and are often touted as very healthy, they are considered problematic because more fructose must be metabolized, potentially resulting in fatty deposits in the liver, blood, and tissues. However, the fact that agave nectar is high in fructose means it is not insulin dependent for metabolism and is theoretically considered diabetic friendly. Fructose, however, has also been linked to insulin resistance, and in high doses can raise the amount of fats in the blood, which is particularly bad for diabetics.

Too much sugar in any form, beyond our need for fuel, will result in excess being turned into fat, and it is well accepted that too much sugar in the diet can contribute to health problems, including obesity and tooth decay. Sugar is also addictive. The more you have, the more you want. Have you noticed how easy it is to put a little more sugar in your tea or coffee over time and then realize you need to scale it back? Scientific evidence points to sugars having similar effects on the brain and similar withdrawal patterns as painkilling drugs, particularly opioids such as morphine.

The main nutritional concern about certain forms of sugar (table sugar, high fructose corn syrup, fruit juice concentrates) is the lack of nutrition and large amount of calories. These forms of sweeteners are considered "empty calories"; they are also highly processed and very acid forming, depleting minerals, particularly calcium from our bones. Although limiting sweeteners is a good thing, we don't want to avoid sweet things altogether; they are an efficient energy source, and sweet foods are simply joyful to taste. Ideally sweet foods consumed should also contain fiber such as that in fruit and vegetables.

For green smoothies, I recommend the following natural sweeteners when you need more sweetness than the fruit in the smoothie provides. I chose them for having either low or no calories, for their balance of glucose and fructose, or for the nutrients they contain. All should be used in small quantities, just enough to do the job.

Stevia A plant whose leaves are at least 250 times sweeter than sugar and with zero calories, stevia can be bought in leaf, powder, or tablet form. Although the best choice for avoiding calories, stevia doesn't taste as pleasant as sugars or syrups.

Xylitol A sugar alcohol derived from the fiber of various plants such as corn and birch, xylitol is slow to convert to glucose in the body. Xylitol keeps blood sugar levels from spiking and thus is a good choice for diabetics. It tastes like sugar but has fewer calories. It has antibacterial properties and assists the transport of calcium in the body, so it is great for preventing tooth decay and for the maintenance of tooth enamel. However, consuming large amounts of xylitol may cause stomach upsets with gas, bloating, and diarrhea.

Raw honey The best choice is unheated and unfiltered raw honey, which is full of substances with amazing nutrients: enzymes, vitamins, minerals, pollens, propolis (resinous material from tree buds that bees use to seal honeycombs), and more. If you can't find the honey I recommend, opt for organic raw honey, meaning it hasn't been heated above the nutrient-destroying temperature of 118°F (48°C).

Maple syrup Although this sap from maple trees is heat treated, it has a good fructose-glucose ratio and is high in vitamins and minerals, particularly potassium and calcium. Also, its taste is sensational!

Dried fruits like sultanas, raisins and dates These very sweet dried fruits can be soaked overnight to plump them up, making them easier to blend.

Agave nectar Since agave nectar is very high-fructose, be sure to use only reputable brands that produce the sweet, mineral-rich syrup without chemicals and are raw, i.e. at low temperatures to preserve enzymes. I use only wild maguey (salmiana variety) agave from the Australian company, Loving Earth. It is certified organic, and organically processed at low temperatures. It contains 70 to 75 percent fructose unlike the Weber blue variety, which can have fructose levels as high as 90 percent. In the United States, an equivalent quality agave to Loving Earth is Xagave.

Rapadura sugar Rapadura, panela, and sucanat are all marketed as types of evaporated sugar cane juice, but rapadura is heated at lower temperatures to retain more vitamins and minerals such as iron. Rapadura is almost truly "raw" sugar, unlike the product mass marketed as raw sugar; that sugar has been heat treated, has little nutrient value, and is barely better than white sugar, which has no nutrient value at all.

Coconut sugar Jaggery or palm sugars, including coconut sugar, are boiled-down flower bud sap and can be found in a block or ground into granules. Although not raw, this type of sugar is mineral rich.

FAQs

What do I use for low-calorie sweeteners?
Stevia and xylitol

Which are the low-GI sweeteners?
Stevia, xylitol, and agave nectar

Which sweeteners are minimally processed?
Organic dried fruits, raw honey, maple syrup, and stevia leaves

Which sweeteners are best for nutrition?
Wild raw honey, dried fruits, raw dark agave nectar, maple syrup, rapadura sugar, and coconut sugar

Which sweetener is the most nutritious?
Wild raw honey

The Importance of Variety

Getting a variety of greens can be challenging when drinking green smoothies on a regular basis. It's easy to stick to the same two or three greens out of convenience and taste preference. I know some people who have never used anything but spinach!

So what happens when you eat a lot of the same thing? First, it's boring! Second, you limit your assimilation of a wide variety of nutrients, and, third, there are chemical-based plant defenses that may create havoc in the form of food intolerances. You may experience an aversion to the food for no apparent reason, or the food may start to make you feel bloated, nauseous, or headachy.

In nature, plants have many defense systems to ensure survival of the species against the herbivores (plant eaters) that love to eat them. Humans are largely unaware of this complex system of mechanical and chemical defenses, as harvests are always available to us at our convenience in supermarkets. Some plant defenses are mechanical, for example, slippery or spiky leaves or stems, aimed primarily at insects and grazing animals. Other defenses are chemical, deterring animals from consuming too much; oxalates, terpenoids, tannins, alkaloids, saponins, and lectins are among the chemicals found in plants, especially greens. We need variety to maximize nutrition and minimize the adverse effects of these secondary metabolites, or plant chemicals, which are either beneficial or harmless in small amounts but problematic in large quantities. This system is part of a concept called "plant defence against herbivory." It exists to protect plant species from being eliminated.

In the wild, animals graze and browse on a variety of plants, a mutually beneficial arrangement for both plants and animals, as plants are not depleted and animals consume an assortment of nutrients. In human dietary terms, "grazing" refers to eating six small meals daily as a theoretical means of maintaining metabolism and blood sugar. In agricultural terms, grazing refers to an herbivore (plant eater) feeding on low lying vegetation and grasses, particularly skimming off the tender shoots and leaves in a way that doesn't harm the plant, still allowing it to regenerate and reproduce. Similarly, "browsing" is a term to describe how an herbivore feeds on fruits, leaves, and shoots of higher growing and usually woody plants like shrubs and trees (e.g., goats are browsers and cattle are grazers). As humans, we don't live in the wild and we are creatures of habit, so it's a challenge to eat a wide variety of foods, particularly greens. When eating multiple handfuls or bunches of greens daily, as is the case when regularly consuming green smoothies, it is vital that you graze on a variety of greens: as much variety as is practical, seasonal, and available.

The topic of rotating greens typically centers on the concept of avoiding the accumulation of alkaloids, with the avoidance of too much oxalate being the hot topic. Oxalate is present in many foods, including greens, particularly spinach and Swiss chard. However, oxalates aren't alkaloids. Alkaloids are nitrogen-based substances that have pharmacological effects on humans and animals. Oxalates, nitrates, and phytates are categorized as chelating poisons. Chelation is a reaction in which molecules bind to minerals. Chelation is used therapeutically for heavy-metal and radiation poisoning using substances like chlorophyll-rich chlorella or EDTA. In these instances, the chelation process removes the heavy metal that is acting as a poison to the body. Chelating poisons on the other hand, can bind to beneficial nutrients like zinc, iron, magnesium, and calcium and remove them from the body via the urine. Calling oxalates a poison might be extreme, but you could say they are a chelating nuisance.

Nitrates can accumulate in plants that are treated with nitrogen-based fertilizers. Phytates primarily exist in the hulls of nuts, seeds, and legumes. Oxalates are well known to be in the leaves of rhubarb, and we have been raised to believe they are extremely poisonous; however, we would need to eat multiple leaves to make us sick. The unpleasant taste would limit that happening—a perfect example of a plant defense mechanism.

Interestingly, lamb's-quarters contain up to 30 times more oxalate than rhubarb leaves. Other high-oxalate foods include beets, buckwheat, cacao, celery, citrus peel, collards, concord grapes, dandelion greens, dried figs, kale, kiwi fruit, lentil sprouts, nuts, oats, parsley, purslane, seeds (especially sesame), sorrel, spinach, star fruit, Swiss chard, and turnip greens. High-oxalate foods not likely to be used in green smoothies include beer, chickpeas, popcorn, soybeans, spelt, tea, and wheat.

Low-oxalate foods that are green smoothie friendly include apples, avocados, berries, lemons, lime juice, and melon.

The concern over oxalate is its nature to bind to minerals, particularly calcium, potentially resulting in calcium deficiency or kidney stones. Many foods high in oxalate are also high in calcium, which may offset the deficiency concern. Various factors influence kidney stones. Calcium oxalate is just one type of stone formation; the body manufactures its own calcium oxalate, and stone formation is linked to a diet low in fiber, greens, complex carbs, and water and high in sugar, refined carbs, and meat. The latter is an acid-forming diet, which fits with the observation of stone formation more frequently occurring in acidic urine. Calcium is an alkaline mineral, after all, so perhaps it's an unfortunate side effect of trying to regain pH balance.

The oxalate argument may seem complex, but we know that oxalated are abundant in nature and not just in greens like spinach and Swiss chard. Oxalates will give you that "spinach teeth" sensation when eating them and may cause some nausea if you consume them too often. The bottom line is, eating a variety of greens, a mixture of high- and low-oxalate foods, and a predominantly alkaline-forming diet will make you less likely to develop kidney stones or a calcium deficiency in the first place.

In addition to chelating poisons are various subgroups of chemical defenses, including nitrogen compounds (alkaloids, cyanogenic glycosides, and glucosinolates), terpenoids, phenolic compounds, certain proteins, and some minerals.

Alkaloids are derived from amino acids (the building blocks of protein) and include pharmacological substances such as quinine, caffeine, and nicotine. Alkaloids have a variety of potentially problematic effects, including inhibition of enzyme activity, alteration of fat or carbohydrate storage, interference with DNA repair, and damage to cell walls.

The effects of cyanogenic glycosides and glucosinolates take hold once the cell walls containing them are broken, releasing substances that have a repellent odor or unpleasant taste or may upset the gastrointestinal tract once ingested. An example of a glycoside is saponin, which has foaming characteristics and tastes bitter. Some plant saponins, such as in oats and spinach, are considered beneficial because they assist the absorption of silica and calcium. Saponins are also present in alfalfa, chickweed, quinoa, asparagus, and daisies. They can be poisonous to animals, but to humans a welcome side effect may be cholesterol reduction.

Terpenoids include elements of volatile essential oils such as menthol, citronella, linalool, and limonene. Menthol is found in mint varieties, tarragon, rose geranium, and basil. Limonene is present primarily in lemon essential oil and also in other citrus fruits and oils, fennel, cardamom, mint, and thyme. Both report antibacterial, antiseptic, and anti-inflammatory effects when consumed in small quantities; they can be allergenic, sedating, and irritating in larger amounts.

Tannins, phenolic compounds found in great abundance in the plant kingdom, give you that dry, puckery feeling in your mouth when you eat them. They protect plants from frost and microbial attack, and their bitter, astringent taste keeps animals from overgrazing. Tannins are also metal chelators, particularly of non-heme iron, which is plant-based iron (versus heme iron in animal flesh), interfering with its assimilation by the body. Tannins also bind to proteins, which affects absorption if the tannins are eaten in large quantities. The compounds are present in berries, cacao, coffee, pecans, pomegranates, red legumes, tea, unripe fruit (especially hachiya persimmons, walnuts, wine, and some herbs and spices).

Tryptophan is an amino acid that in small doses has reported benefits on mood and sleep, though in high doses it may promote tumors. It occurs naturally in almonds, beans, chicory, evening primrose, mung beans, spinach, sunflowers, watercress, pumpkinseeds, and purslane, all of which may have a place in green smoothies in leaf, sprout, or nut or seed milk form.

Selenium is a mineral that in low doses has a huge range of beneficial effects, including being a powerful antioxidant. In higher doses it is toxic to humans and animals. The immune-boosting herb astragalus is an example of a seleniferous plant whose bitter taste and strong odor deters herbivores. Other naturally occurring sources of selenium are Brazil nuts, thyme, clover, peppermint, skullcap, almonds, cabbage, cashews, buckwheat, and pumpkinseeds, all of which may have a place in green smoothies in leaf, tea, sprout, or nut or seed milk form.

Not all plant defenses need to be overcome by variety. Adaptations can be mechanical, behavioral, or biochemical. Insects adapt to woody and silica-rich plant stems by developing stronger claws and jaws. As a biochemical adaptation, some herbivores have enzymes such as mixed function oxidases (MFOs) they use to detoxify or reduce the effectiveness of some plant chemicals. Behaviorally, animals learn that newer leaves, certain parts of leaves, or timing of seasons dictate the dosage of plant chemicals consumed.

Humans have adapted by cooking, soaking, sprouting, fermenting, or blending to make some plants digestible or palatable or to maximize nutrient absorption. For instance, the cell walls of some plants consist of indigestible, insoluble fiber. Those cell walls must be disrupted—by cooking, blending, or a lot of chewing—to release the nutrients locked inside.

The starch in grains, legumes, and starchy tubers like potatoes requires cooking for digestibility. The cooking process changes the structure by gelatinizing the starch and neutralizing enzyme inhibitors. Secondary metabolites, or anti-nutrients, in protein-rich foods like nuts, seeds, and legumes include protease inhibitors, tannins, saponins, lectins, and phytates. Cooking destroys these substances, allowing better access to the protein. On the flip side, cooking itself denatures or changes the natural qualities of protein. Soaking, sprouting, and fermenting are also methods to reduce these anti-nutrients to improve digestion and make nutrients more available.

For green smoothies, the anti-nutrient content of nuts and seeds is relevant if you use them either whole or as milk. Soaking nuts and seeds for as little as 4 hours or overnight will affect the anti-nutrient content, such as the reduction of phytates making minerals available in a form that is more easily absorbed into the bloodstream, and the disarming of enzyme inhibitors aids digestion. The reason such anti-nutrients exists in nuts and seeds is to prevent them from growing while in storage. Instead they remain dormant until "activated" by water. If you see nuts or seeds sold as "activated," it means that they have been soaked and dehydrated again, making them healthier yet still crunchy.

To minimize problems with the plants' chemical defenses and to maximize nutrition and enthusiasm about drinking green smoothies, aim to rotate through at least six different greens on a regular basis. Try to have three types of greens washed and ready to use in the refrigerator, and change your selection each week. Also challenge yourself to introduce more obscure greens, herbs, sprouts, and edible weeds as you become more experienced. You will be surprised at what works. Radish leaves are surprisingly mild tasting, and fennel tops are simply amazing. These won't ever be daily or even weekly options the way spinach and kale probably will, but experiment with what is growing in your garden and with items you might normally throw away.

Be aware that all plant foods, even fruits, contain secondary metabolites to some degree, so variety is important in your diet generally and in your choice of green smoothie ingredients, including greens, fruits, nuts, and seeds. Eating with the seasons is the best way of encouraging variety to avoid potential digestive problems and ensure a broad spectrum of nutrients. Be sure to check out my recipes for spring smoothies (page 108), summer smoothies (page 113), autumn smoothies (page 119), and winter smoothies (page 125).

Superfoods in Green Smoothies

There is no consensus among experts about whether or not we should add superfoods to our diets and this includes ambiguity on whether we should include them in green smoothies. David Wolfe is famous in the raw food world for his love of superfoods, though even he doesn't live on them alone.

There is no standard, regulated definition of the term "superfood," but the consensus is that superfoods are super-nutritious and contain not just one or a few nutrients but many. You'll see the term used for everything from true superfoods like cacao, maca, noni, and AFA blue-green algae to less credible items such as ice cream and bacon.

The term "functional food," also unregulated, refers to aspects of foods that serve particular functions to promote health or prevent disease. Generally these are processed foods that claim, for example, to be high in fiber or fortified with minerals such as folic acid or iodine. Usually the food producer has added an ingredient that was lacking in the soil, such as iodine, or was lost by processing the product and stripping it of fiber and many vitamins and minerals, such as occurs when processing whole wheat to make white bread.

Processed functional foods are not super-nutritious; nutrition has merely been added to nutrient-poor food. However, natural, unprocessed functional foods may be particularly rich in a specific ingredient or two, making them very beneficial to the diet. Some people might argue that a natural, unprocessed functional food is a superfood.

When someone consumes a diet that eliminates certain foods such as dairy and meat, inevitably well-meaning and less knowledgeable friends and family members will raise concerns. The classic concern is whether the person is getting enough calcium, protein, vitamin B12, and iron. What the friends and family members don't know is that nutrient deficiencies are just as prevalent among people eating meat and dairy as among those who don't. Ultimately, it comes down to how nutritious a diet is overall and how well the nutrients are absorbed. There are concerns with everyone's diet when it come to the consumption of good fats such as omega-3s, magnesium, iodine, zinc, B vitamins, and fiber.

Omega-3 fats are essential for the joints, brain, and heart, and we need an alternative to eating at least six servings of fish every day to get enough. Magnesium and iodine are extremely deficient in most soils and thus in plants growing in those soils. Magnesium, iodine, zinc, and B vitamins are depleted in the body by stress, and we live in a stressful world. Without these nutrients, physical, mental, and hormonal health suffer. Fiber is essential for removal of bad cholesterol and to keep the bowels moving, yet cholesterol-lowering drugs and constipation are prevalent in our society.

It is clear we are in desperate need of a variety of nutrients from a variety of sources.

Not all people have access to the very best organic, freshly picked produce whenever they want it. Many feel that if they are not getting all the nutrients they need, or if they need extra of something to perform a particular function, then they can take a supplement. For some, this is in the form of tablets, but I prefer to use plant-based superfoods and natural functional foods that deliver extra nutrients. The following are excellent examples of green smoothie–friendly superfoods to boost nutrition.

Chia Seeds

The Aztecs so revered chia seeds that they used them as currency. Today we hold chia in high regard as the plant with the highest amount of omega-3 fats. These are essential fatty acids (EFAs), meaning they must be supplied in food. EFAs are essential for the nervous system, brain, cardiovascular system, skin, and joints.

Unlike flax and fish, which also contain omega-3s, chia is very stable due to its high antioxidant value. Ground flax seeds and flax oil must be kept strictly refrigerated and used very quickly (in 1 to 2 weeks) or they go rancid. Chia has similar to slightly greater antioxidant strength than blueberries, and black chia seeds have approximately 25 percent more antioxidants than white.

Chia is low on the glycemic index (see page 56), gluten free, and jam packed with nutrients, including a complete amino acid profile. This means it contains all eight essential amino acids, which is rare in plants. Our bodies can't manufacture these amino acids, so they must be provided in food. Amino acids are the building blocks of protein that form tissues like muscles and skin, and they help create enzymes. Chia contains up to 23 percent protein and 18 amino acids including tryptophan, important for relaxation and sleep, and tyrosine, key for mood and thyroid health.

Rich in calcium, iron, magnesium, zinc, potassium, phosphorus, and A, B, and C vitamins, chia also consists of 37 percent fiber, including insoluble, which keeps us regular, and soluble, which bulks and softens stools and helps remove bad cholesterol (LDL) from the body.

Chia seeds form a tasteless gel in liquid just as flax seeds do, but chia will go completely soft. The seeds are tiny and break down easily; they can be ground into a powder in the blender prior to adding the rest of the ingredients or they can be added whole. If left to sit, 1 to 2 tablespoons of chia will thicken a smoothie, so drink it immediately if you want the smoothie consistency to remain the same, or let it thicken if desired. If 2 to 4 tablespoons of chia is used, the smoothie will turn into a pudding consistency that can be eaten with a spoon.

Chia experts recommend that 1 tablespoon daily is ideal to boost an already nutritious diet. Higher amounts (2 to 4 tablespoons) can be used for extra nutrition, for extra fiber, and for feelings of fullness if used as an appetite suppressant. Higher amounts will have a laxative effect on the bowel, which may be beneficial to some people, but others should take with caution.

Micro-algae

Spirulina, chlorella, AFA (*Alphanizemenon flos-aquae*), and MPP (marine phytoplankton) are all single-cell organisms that have similar nutritional profiles though with some key differences. They all boast a similar abundance of vitamins, minerals, enzymes, 60 percent or more protein, all essential amino acids, essential fatty acids, RNA, DNA, and antioxidant pigments (primarily chlorophyll). Nutritionist Dr. Gillian McKeith and superfood expert David Wolfe have researched micro-algae extensively and report that they have immune-boosting, antibacterial, antifungal, and antiviral properties. In addition, micro-algae improve mental capacity, fight cancer, detoxify, act as anti-inflammatory agents, are blood building, and are highly absorbable (the body can assimilate 90 to 100 percent).

Chlorella and spirulina are cultivated in fresh water ponds and lakes. AFA is wild and harvested only from the cold waters of Klamath Lake in Oregon. MPP is a salt water–based micro-algae found in oceans and seas.

Chlorella is the richest source of chlorophyll, which is similar to hemoglobin in human blood; chlorophyll is based on magnesium and hemoglobin on iron. Chlorella is considered the best of the micro-algae for detoxifying the body of heavy metals and offering protection against radiation.

Spirulina, AFA, and some chlorella strains contain the blue pigment phycocyanin, which is an antioxidant, is blood building along with chlorophyll, and enhances stem cells. Because they contain both the blue pigment and the green chlorophyll pigment, these micro-algae are often termed blue-green algae. They all also have a variety of red, orange, and yellow antioxidant pigments, which are in the cancer-fighting group of carotenoids.

Although all micro-algae are protein rich, spirulina is the richest with around 70 percent protein. Slightly lower in overall nutrients than the other micro-algae, spirulina is also considered the easiest to digest. Chlorella is the most difficult to digest because, unlike the others, it has a tough cell wall and thus supplements must be cell-wall broken to be effective. Also, some people lack the right enzyme to metabolize chlorella. Japanese research reports that spirulina and chlorella beneficially enhance the reproduction of *Lactobacillus* bacteria in the stomach.

Unique to AFA is the substance PEA (phenylethylamine), sometimes called the "love chemical," which raises dopamine levels. Also present in cacao, PEA aids concentration and improves attitude and well-being. Dopamine deficiency is associated with depression as well as Parkinson's disease.

Each of these amazing micro-algae contains essential fatty acids (EFAs), though the salient types differ in each. Spirulina contains a lot of an omega-6 called gamma-linolenic acid (GLA): The amount is second only to that in mother's milk. GLA is anti-inflammatory and good for allergies. AFA primarily contains omega-3s in the form of alpha-linolenic acid (ALA) and to a lesser extent omega-6s as linoleic acid (LA) and GLA. MPP contains ALA and the omega-3s eicosapentaenoic acid (EPA) and docosahexaenoic acid (DHA). Chlorella is rich in ALA.

The omega-3s EPA and DHA are otherwise found only in seafood. Plants contain ALA, which is converted to EPA and DHA in the body—although this process requires good body chemistry and the presence of B vitamins and magnesium. Consuming MPP is a good insurance policy for vegans and vegetarians and anyone not eating a lot of seafood, to ensure sufficient EPA and DHA is supplied for brain, eye, and reproductive health. Coconut oil can also assist with the conversion of ALA to DHA, so it's a great idea to include coconut oil in green smoothies when also using plant-based ALA such as that in flax and chia, and algae-based ALA in micro-algae.

Supplementing with micro-algae appears very attractive based on their attributes, and it's clear each provides unique benefits:

Spirulina for allergies, digestibility, high protein content, and improved reproduction of probiotics in the gut. Children minimally or not breast-fed can benefit from the GLA in spirulina. I recommend In-Liven Fermented Probiotic Superfood, which contains spirulina and probiotics.

AFA for PEA, which will improve mood and for extra nutrients generally. AFA is also a truly wild food. I recommend E3Live or Ancient Sun Crystal Manna.

MPP for additional nutrition (especially minerals), DHA, and EPA. I recommend Ocean's Alive or Longevity MPP.

Chlorella for heavy-metal detoxification and radiation protection. Look for products that are "cell-wall broken" and cold processed.

Bee Pollen

An amazing source of nutrients, bee pollen cannot be produced synthetically. Bees collect pollen from flowers; the pollen mixes with honey brought from the hive and is stored in pockets in the bee's legs, where it's packed down to form a granule. Bee pollen is taken back to the hive as a food source for the bees; it is rich in protein (25 to 40 percent), amino acids, hormones, fats, carbohydrates, lecithin, nucleic acids, all B vitamins, and other vitamins. Bee pollen is considered one of the most complete foods in nature. It is alkaline, energizing, high in antioxidants, and easily

In-Liven Fermented Probiotic Superfood

If I could take one food or superfood to a desert island, it would be In-Liven. It has been instrumental in helping me conquer candida in my gut, and I never go a day without it. I add 1 teaspoon to my smoothie every day, and every 3 months I take it 3 times a day for a week.

In-Liven is the result of more than 20 years of research and development. It is a raw, certified-organic, fermented, probiotic superfood, acting as a four-in-one supplement:

1. A probiotic formula containing all 13 *Lactobacillus*-friendly bacteria and 2 strains of beneficial *Saccharomyces* yeasts.

2. A prebiotic formula as it also contains malt liquid and molasses as an ongoing food source for the bacteria.

3. A digestive enzymes formula when taken before meals (enzymes from the bacteria and the living whole foods in the formula).

4. A nutritional formula containing 20 amino acids, including the 8 essentials, as well as vitamins, minerals, and trace elements from spirulina, grass powders, vegetables, and grains.

The 26 whole foods in In-Liven are pre-digested and fermented by the *Lactobacillus* bacteria for 3 weeks before bottling. The bacteria completely break down the plant cell walls, allowing 100 percent availability of nutrients (versus about 20 percent when you ingest the same foods yourself).

The *Lactobacillus* in In-Liven have been bred to withstand many conditions such as high heat, extreme cold, acid, pollution, and ascorbic acid. This means that only the fittest bacteria survive and are used. They don't require refrigeration, and they are able to journey though the human digestive tract to where they are needed in the bowel.

In-Liven contains both *Lactobacillus* and spirulina. We know that spirulina is the easiest of the micro-algae to digest, and it aids the reproduction of *Lactobacillus* bacteria in the gut.

absorbed. It improves athletic performance, aids fertility, and can help allergies by reducing the production of histamines.

Bee pollen can produce allergenic reactions in some people and so must be used with caution. We started using it in our smoothies to assist with my husband's hay fever. We began with ⅛ teaspoon and built up slowly to 1 teaspoon. I know other people take bigger doses, but we stopped at this amount out of respect for the bees!

Raw Cacao

The raw form of what is known conventionally as chocolate or cocoa is referred to as cacao. Its botanical name is *Theobroma cacao*, the first part of the name meaning "food of the gods." Like the Aztecs did with chia, Mayans so revered cacao beans that they used them as currency instead of gold. Originally eaten in its raw and bitter state in South America, cacao ultimately became a delicacy heated and mixed with sugar and milk when it reached Europe.

Cacao contains literally hundreds of nutrients and phytochemicals, ranging from abundant levels of antioxidant substances to small amounts of trace minerals. In its raw form, cacao has one of the highest antioxidant values of any plant in the world (similar to the Amazonian acai berry and second only to the Patagonian maqui berry).

The cacao bean is low in fat. Containing 50 percent fat, cacao is rich in omega-6 essential fatty acids. Cacao is high in soluble fiber, so it's gut and cholesterol friendly. It is rich in minerals, particularly magnesium, frequently deficient in people's diets but important for bone and cardiovascular health. Cacao is also a good source of iron for the blood, manganese to provide a necessary enzyme activator, chromium for blood sugar, and zinc for immunity, mental health, and reproduction.

Cacao contains minute amounts of caffeine, though it does have larger amounts of theobromine, a compound resembling caffeine. Some people report that they feel stimulated by cacao but others don't; if you are the first camp, you'll be wise not to consume cacao in the evening.

The main reason people consume cacao and are so attracted to it is because it makes them feel good. Cacao is full of feel-good substances such as PEA (phenylethylamine), the "love chemical" that is found in wild blue-green AFA algae, and it also acts as an appetite suppressant. As well, cacao contains anandamide, sometimes called the "bliss chemical," which the body produces after vigorous exercise. Another substance in cacao is tryptophan, the precursor to serotonin, an antidepressant chemical produced by the pineal gland in the brain and in the stomach. With such feel-good chemicals in our system after consuming cacao, it's little wonder people fall in love with it and crave it when feeling low.

Antioxidants

Oxidation, degradation, corrosion, tarnishing, rusting—they all describe the breakdown of a substance due to a chemical reaction with its surroundings. The classic example is iron rusting into iron oxide when exposed to water. Because nature always seeks balance, or homeostasis, and energy conservation, the rusting of iron is nature's way of returning the manufactured form of iron to the more stable state that exists in nature.

Antioxidant refers to anti-oxidation. "Oxidation" is a term used in chemistry to describe the net loss of electrons, which are tiny particles within an atom that have a negative charge (protons are positive). The opposite is "reduction," which describes the net gain of electrons.

Nature's desire for homeostasis results in redox (REDuction – OXidation) reactions, which occur continuously in nature and in the human body. For example, photosynthesis in plants involves the conversion of carbon dioxide, water, and sunlight energy into sugars that are stored in plants and the release of oxygen as a by-product. Human cellular respiration involves the opposite reaction, the conversion of glucose and oxygen into carbon dioxide, water, and energy. Each reaction has two parts, one part an oxidation reaction and one part a reduction reaction. Ideally, any free electron that detaches itself will reattach immediately. If it doesn't, it becomes a free radical. Free radicals are unstable and seek out attachment to anything that can give them electrical balance. In the best-case scenarios, attachment occurs within a redox reaction or free radicals attach to and are neutralized by antioxidant substances. If neither scenario happens, then free radicals attach themselves to any surface they can, which can lead to cellular damage and a cascade of destruction, including cell mutation.

Degradation due to oxidation occurs not only in metals but also in the human body. Free radical formation in the body can be accelerated by external influences such as tobacco smoke, toxins, pollution, stress, and poor eating habits. Scientists have known for decades that free radical damage can be linked to cancer, cardiovascular disease, rheumatoid arthritis, diabetes, and age-related diseases.

A diet rich in antioxidants, which exist in plants and algae, is the ideal army to fight free radicals. Antioxidant substances include vitamins A, C, and E as well as selenium, coenzyme Q10, glutathione, flavonoids, polyphenols, and plant pigments such as chlorophyll and carotenoids.

ORAC (Oxygen Radical Absorbance Capacity) is a standardized measurement of the total antioxidant power of a food. Antioxidant power is the ability to neutralize free radicals. It is well known that many of the world's developed countries have nutrient-deficient soils, particularly Australia, where I live. It is estimated that 70 percent of the population of developed countries is micronutrient malnourished. Thus nutritionists recommend consuming at least seven servings of fruits and vegetables per day, which will supply sufficient antioxidant activity in the body to reduce free radical damage. Seven servings of fruits or vegetables provide around 3,500 ORAC units, but my problem with this calculation is that not all fruits and vegetables are created equal. Seven servings of iceberg lettuce are different from seven servings of fresh berries. Furthermore, the freshness of a food as well as whether it is organic influences its nutrition level.

Personally, I aim to eat an antioxidant-rich diet that emphasizes such foods as dark greens, berries, algae, brightly colored vegetables, chia seeds, coconut, and cacao. I add a food-based powder called Berry Radical, a raw, certified-organic, antioxidant superfood with a very high ORAC score. It is a potent combination of nine of the world's most effective antioxidant superfoods: raw cacao, olive juice extract, coffee fruit extract, and freeze-dried fruits and berries, including pomegranate, goji berries, strawberries, blueberries, acai berries, and raspberries. One teaspoon serving of Berry Radical contains over 4,000 ORAC units. Unlike many antioxidant products on the market, Berry Radical comes in powder form and so has no need for preservatives. A heaping teaspoon in a green smoothie provides a great start to the day. It can also be made into a delicious and a very healthy hot chocolate by mixing a teaspoon with warm milk and added sweetener.

Hemp Seeds

Hemp seeds, or the seeds of the plant *Cannabis sativa*, are said to contain all the essential amino acids and essential fatty acids. The seeds are soft and easy to digest raw, and the essential fatty acids omega-6 and omega-3 are in the ideal ratio of 3:1. The omega-6s are linoleic acid (LA) and the anti-inflammatory gamma-linolenic acid (GLA); omega-3s are in the form of alpha-linolenic acid (ALA). Hemp seeds are rich in chlorophyll, magnesium, potassium, sulfur, calcium, iron, phosphorus, and vitamins A, B, and C. They also consist of 35 percent fiber, which includes both soluble and insoluble.

The only countries in the world where foodstuffs made from hemp seeds and hemp oil are illegal for human consumption are in Australia and New Zealand. This is despite the recommendation a few years back by the Food Standards Australia New Zealand (FSANZ) that the prohibition be removed. However, state ministers and government heads rejected the proposal, determining in their wisdom, that there would be law enforcement difficulties distinguishing between high-THC *Cannabis sativa* (marijuana) and low-THC *sativa* (hemp), which cannot get you high. They also believed that the use of industrial hemp in food may send a confused message to consumers about the acceptability and safety of hemp. Sounds a bit silly to me and a bit backward, and I am saying this about my own country!

I did get some hemp seeds when I was recently in the UK and they are just fantastic! They are a great way to make green smoothies beautifully creamy, especially if you don't want to use bananas or don't have any on hand. In addition to adding them to my smoothies, I sprinkled them on salads and ate them by the spoonful.

Deep Green Alkalising Superfood

Since using fresh, raw greens is the point of green smoothies, the idea of adding green powder is controversial. For some, a green powder is what makes a green smoothie green, but for purists, it's cheating.

I believe a green powder has its place under certain circumstances:

- You have run out of greens—this does happen!
- The variety of greens available to you is limited.
- You have a brand that is reputable and of excellent quality.
- You're traveling or staying with friends or family where having a smoothie may not be an option. Instead you can mix a green powder into juice or water.

My choice is Deep Green Alkalising Superfood.

Deep Green is raw and vegan, and contains certified-organic blue-green algae, green grass juices, and leafy green vegetables. Specifically, it has spirulina, cold-temperature dried alfalfa, barley, kamut, oat, and wheat grass juice powders, and freeze-dried pure spinach, kale, parsley, collard, and nettle powders.

Having this variety in a formulation is great, as you get key nutrients from specific greens. For example, you'll get SOD (the antioxidant superoxide dismutase) from barley, chromium from nettles, tyrosine and GLA from spirulina, vitamin C and beta-carotene from parsley, more than 40 bioflavanoids from alfalfa, isothiocyanates and vitamin K from kale, complete vitamins and essential amino acids from wheat grass, folic acid and manganese from spinach, selenium and zinc from kamut, iron and calcium from oats, and four cancer-fighting glucosinolates from collards. How amazing are greens!

Most grass powders on the market use processing methods that involve drying with high heat and oxygen exposure, which damage and denature enzymes and nutrients. Furthermore, many grass juice powders are diluted with the food additive maltodextrin and other cheap fillers like rice bran, flax seed, or legumes.

Unlike horses and cows, humans can't digest the tough cell walls in grasses, which means we miss out on the nutrients locked inside them. Grass juices make these nutrients more easily absorbed in the stomach and Deep Green only includes grass juice powders in the formula.

Just 1 teaspoon of concentrated, dense Deep Green powder is equivalent to over 2 fluid ounces (60 mL) of fresh green juice. Add it to a smoothie or stir it into water or juice.

There are many more superfoods that can be added to smoothies and listing them all could be a book on its own. If you wish to find out more, please check the Appendix on page 234 for suggested books and websites about superfoods.

PART TWO

Green Smoothie Recipes

Given the variation of produce around the world and the huge number of green smoothie recipes available, I have arranged all of the recipes in this book into categories. For those passionate about eating with the seasons, there are chapters for spring, summer, autumn, and winter. There are recipes for green smoothies for children, recipes for superfood fans, for those with specific concerns like weight loss or cardiovascular health, and many more.

Here are a few guidelines for using these recipes:

Recipes make enough for about 1 quart (1 liter) of green smoothie unless otherwise stated. This is enough for about 2 servings.

Specific types and amounts of greens are not given unless a particular flavor or nutritional benefit is desired. If just "greens" is stated, use whatever raw, leafy greens you like, and as much or as little as you like. If you're new to green smoothies, start with a small handful of mild greens, like spinach, and with time you will naturally increase the amount and variety you use.

Use good quality ripe fruit and fresh water. Unripe fruit will make your smoothie taste unpleasant. Try to buy organic produce and, if possible, from farmer's markets, where the produce will be fresher. I also recommend using the best source of water possible and at a minimum, filtered tap water.

Slice or break fruit into appropriately sized pieces for your blender. The larger and more powerful the blender, the larger pieces it will handle, such as quartered apples. Less expensive or small blenders will require smaller pieces of fruit.

It's assumed that fruit such as bananas, mangoes, melons, and papaya are peeled and that stone fruit such as cherries have pits removed. Apples don't need to be cored; however, pears do.

Specific blending times are not given, as this will vary among blenders. You will get to know your own blender well and will learn to know when your smoothie is ready. (For more information on different blenders, see page 43.)

If your blender tends to make your smoothie warm, use ice cubes in place of some of the liquid in a recipe, or use some frozen fruit in place of fresh fruit. Ice blended through a smoothie can also aid the breakdown of particularly fibrous ingredients like whole lemons and celery, to help create a smoother smoothie. Be careful not to regularly consume green smoothies that are very cold to avoid potential digestive strain.

Be sure to check the smoothie's flavor and consistency before serving since ingredients will vary in size, texture, and sweetness.

- If it's too thick, add more water or other liquid.
- If it's too thin, add more fruit or 1–2 tablespoons of chia seeds.
- If it's too tart, add sweetener, like stevia, xylitol, agave, honey, dates, or maple syrup.
- If it's too bitter, add lemon juice, sweetener, and/or vanilla extract.

As you experiment with making green smoothies, you will realize that some ingredients just don't go well together, like pineapple and cacao, or coconut and tomatoes, but there are seemingly limitless green smoothie possibilities, so you're certain to come upon winning combinations.

All of these green smoothie recipes have been designed with flavor and texture pairing in mind. I hope you enjoy them as much as I do!

To get the ball rolling, here is my daily green smoothie recipe:

Basic Green Smoothie

3 to 4 bananas, or 2 bananas plus 1 cup frozen blueberries

2 teaspoons In-Liven Fermented Probiotic Superfood

1½ cups water

generous amount of greens

1 teaspoon vanilla extract

Blend for 1 to 2 minutes in a high-powered blender and serve in 2 large glasses.

Spring

Spring is a beautiful time of year, as flowers bloom and baby animals are born after the cold of winter passes, but it is a surprisingly limited time for produce.

As gardens are planted for later harvests, earlier spring fruits available include:

- avocados
- blood oranges
- grapefruit
- kumquats
- lemons

- mandarin oranges
- papaya
- star fruit
- tangelos
- Valencia oranges

Later fruit are:

- bananas
- blueberries
- cucumbers
- lychees

- mangoes
- melons
- raspberries
- strawberries

Spring greens include:

- Asian greens
- beet greens
- cabbage
- carrot tops
- cilantro
- lettuce varieties
- mint
- parsley
- pea greens
- spinach
- Swiss chard
- turnip greens
- watercress

What you find in season at the spring market will vary based on where you live. In more moderate climates, such as where I live in Southern Australia, many of these fruits will be readily available, while others may be very hard to find. Use this opportunity to experiment with what is fresh to create your own green smoothies.

Spring Recipes

1 cup red papaya

2 bananas

1½ cups water

greens

1 cup star fruit

½ cup young coconut flesh

1½ cups coconut water

cilantro

2 mangoes

½ teaspoon ground cardamom

1½ cups almond milk

greens

1 cup peeled, seeded lychees

½ cup blueberries

1 banana

1 cup water or nut milk

greens

---

2 bananas

1 cup unhulled strawberries

flesh and zest of 1 lemon

1 cup water or nut milk

mint

cilantro

1½ cups cantaloupe

I cup unhulled strawberries

1 cup water

greens

2½ cups honeydew melon

1 inch fresh ginger

zest of ½ lemon

1 cup water

greens

2½ cups watermelon

1 cup raspberries

1 lime, peeled

greens

---

1 mango

flesh and water of 1 Thai coconut

1 lime, peeled

greens

1 cup unhulled strawberries

1 small pink grapefruit, peeled

mint

greens

---

1 cup papaya

1 orange, peeled

1 lime, peeled

1½ cups orange juice

greens

---

1 cup pink grapefruit, peeled

2 mandarin oranges, peeled

zest and flesh of 1 lemon

½ avocado

greens

sweetener, as needed

---

1 cup whole kumquats

1 apple

1 Lebanese cucumber

1 teaspoon vanilla extract

1 cup water

parsley

---

2 oranges, peeled

1 lime, peeled

½ avocado

1½ cups orange juice

watercress

1 cup cranberries

1 orange, peeled

zest of ½ orange

1½ cups orange juice

greens

Summer

In some parts of the world, it's summer all year round, but in many places it's only for a few too-brief months. Either way, summer is synonymous with luscious, sweet fruits. It is a magical time for green smoothies, and also a great time to buy bulk produce such as mangoes, bananas, and berries, when they are at their best quality and inexpensive at the markets. Freeze what you don't use for later in the year when there's less fresh produce available and you need some extra variety.

Summer fruits include:

- avocados
- apricots
- bananas
- berries (all varieties)
- cucumbers
- grapes
- guava
- lemons
- lychees
- mangoes
- melons
- nectarines
- papaya
- passion fruit
- peaches
- plums
- tomatoes
- Valencia oranges

Summer greens include:

- amaranth
- basil
- celery
- dandelion
- lamb's-quarters
- lettuce varieties
- mint
- nasturtium
- parsley
- sorrel
- strawberry leaves
- Swiss chard
- watercress

Summer Recipes

2 cups apricots

½ teaspoon ground cinnamon

¼ teaspoon ground cardamom

1 teaspoon vanilla extract

1½ cups almond milk

greens

1 cup blueberries

1 large banana

1½ cups of nut milk or water

greens

1½ cups berries

flesh and water of 1 young coconut

small handful of basil leaves

spinach

3½ cups watermelon

1 inch fresh ginger

2 tablespoons chia seeds (optional, for a thicker smoothie)

greens

1 mango

1 banana

1½ cups water

greens

1 cup unhulled strawberries

1 cup frozen unhulled strawberries

1 cup cashew milk

basil

1½ cups red papaya

1 cup inner rib celery leaves

romaine lettuce leaves from the middle of the head

1½ cups water

2 plums

1 peach

1 teaspoon vanilla extract

1½ cups of water or almond milk

greens

1½ cups red or green grapes

2 cups melon (any variety)

greens

1 cup of guava or feijoa (pineapple guava)

flesh and water of 1 young coconut

zest and juice of 1 lemon or lime

greens

I cup unhulled strawberries

2 bananas

1 cup water

handful of mint or other green

---

1 cup pitted cherries

1 banana

1 to 2 tablespoons raw cacao

1½ cups water or nut milk

greens

---

2 bananas

1 cup raspberries

zest of 1 lemon

1½ cups water

greens

2½ cups cantaloupe

1 cup unhulled strawberries

mint

greens

---

3 bananas

2 tablespoons raw cacao

1½ cups water or nut milk

mint

greens

---

1 mango

2 oranges, peeled

1 cup water

greens

passion fruit pulp, to top the finished smoothie

Featured Recipe

Author and "Dream Life Coach" **Joanne Newell** (www.richradiantreal
.com) is a huge fan of green smoothies and has kindly submitted two of
her favorites from her green smoothie e-book, *Rich Radiant Real: The
Green Smoothie Glow.*

BERRY RECHARGE

    2 Medjool dates
    1 orange, peeled
    2 bananas
    2 to 3 cups Swiss chard
    ½ cup raspberries
    ½ cup blackberries
    4 strawberries
    ½ cup grapes
    1 cup water

TROP A GO-GO

    flesh and water of 1 young Thai coconut
    1 mango
    2 bananas
    1 cup water
    1 to 2 cups Swiss chard
    1 cup spinach

---

    2 cups peeled, seeded lychees
    1½ cups almond milk
    mint
    greens

    I cup unhulled strawberries
    1 cup apricots or peaches
    1 cup water
    greens

1 cup blood plums

pulp of 2 passion fruit

½ cup ice cubes

1½ cups almond milk

greens

---

1 cup red papaya

1½ cups tomatoes

1 cup water

½ bunch of basil

pinch of salt

Autumn

Autumn is such a beautiful time of the year as the hot summer transitions to mild sunny days, cool nights, and the spectacular changes in the color of leaves. Autumn is my favorite time of the year, especially when there's often a glut of end-of-season summer produce like strawberries and peaches, while new season fruits like apples and pears make a long-awaited return.

Autumn fruits for green smoothies can make an amazing variety of delicious combinations, including:

- apples
- Asian pears
- avocados
- bananas
- cantaloupe
- cucumbers
- feijoa (pineapple guava)
- figs
- grapes
- guava
- honeydew melons
- kiwifruit
- kumquats
- lemons
- limes
- nectarines
- passion fruit
- peaches
- pears
- persimmons
- plums
- pomegranate
- raspberries
- strawberries
- tomatoes
- Valencia oranges

Autumn greens include:

- Asian greens
- basil
- beet greens
- carrot tops
- celery
- cilantro
- endive
- fennel tops
- kale
- lettuce varieties
- mint
- parsley
- pumpkin leaves
- radish tops
- Swiss chard

Autumn Recipes

4 fresh figs

1 cup raspberries

1½ cups water or nut milk

greens

1 apple

½ avocado

1 teaspoon ground cinnamon

½ teaspoon ground cardamom

1 teaspoon vanilla extract

1½ cups water

greens

3 peaches

½ cup raspberries

1 teaspoon vanilla extract

1½ cups water

greens

4 fresh figs

1½ cups red grapes

½ teaspoon ground cinnamon

1 cup water

greens

2 kiwifruit

½ avocado

2 oranges, peeled

1½ cups water

mint

1½ cups honeydew melon

1 cup green grapes

1 cup water

greens

1½ cups cantaloupe

1 cup raspberries and/or strawberries

1 cup water

greens

3 pears

1 teaspoon ground cinnamon

⅛ teaspoon ground clove

½ teaspoon ground cardamom

1 inch fresh ginger

1 teaspoon vanilla extract

1½ cups almond milk

greens

1 cup ripe (non-astringent) fuyu persimmon flesh

½ avocado

1 cup almond milk

1 cup water

greens

---

1 cup very, very ripe hachiya persimmon flesh

1 lemon (if lots of pith, slice most off)

1 lime, peeled

1 cup ice cubes

½ cup water

greens

sweetener, as needed

---

1 apple

1 cup whole kumquats

flesh and zest of 1 lemon

4 tablespoons hemp seeds or 2 tablespoons walnut oil

½ cup water

1 cup ice cubes

cabbage, kale, or parsley

---

2 Asian pears

1 banana

1½ cups water

greens

flesh of 1 to 2 passion fruit per serving, stirred through the finished smoothies

---

2 bananas

4 passion fruit

1 orange, peeled

1½ cups water

greens

2 to 3 nectarines

flesh of 2 lemons

zest of 1 lemon

1 inch fresh ginger

1½ cups water

greens

sweetener, as needed

2 bananas

1 to 2 peaches

1 teaspoon ground cinnamon

1½ cups water

greens

3 oranges, peeled

juice of 1 large or 2 small pomegranates*

1 cup water or nut milk

parsley

* To juice pomegranates, peel and blend whole, then strain
  through a nut milk bag or cheesecloth.

4 plums

zest of 1 orange

1 teaspoon vanilla extract

1 cup almond milk

1 cup water

greens

3 peaches

3 to 4 fresh figs

½ teaspoon ground cinnamon

1 teaspoon vanilla extract

1½ cups water

greens

2 cups honeydew melon

1 Lebanese cucumber

½ cup ice cubes

mint

greens

1 cup fresh unhulled strawberries

1 cup frozen unhulled strawberries

1 cup cashew milk

basil

spinach

Winter

Winter produce can certainly present a challenge compared with the abundance of summer fruits. But it also can be a time for creativity when it comes to green smoothies.

Ginger and warming spices like cinnamon can be used. Nut milks, ginger, and spices can add a more filling and warming element to a winter green smoothie. By the same token, use of ice and frozen fruit is best avoided given the weather is cold enough as it is!

In winter there is an abundance of citrus available, which can't be a coincidence given our need for nutrients like vitamin C to help ward off coughs and colds. Key winter fruits include:

- apples
- Asian pears
- avocados
- grapefruit
- kiwifruit
- lemons
- limes
- mandarin oranges
- navel oranges
- papaya
- pears
- persimmons
- pineapple
- pomegranates
- tamarillos
- tangelos

Nutritious winter greens include:

- Asian greens
- beet greens
- cabbage
- carrot tops
- celery
- cilantro
- fennel tops
- kale
- parsley
- radish tops
- spinach
- Swiss chard
- turnip greens

Winter Recipes

2 bananas

zest of 1 lemon

flesh of 2 lemons

1½ cups water

parsley

....

1 apple

1 banana

1 celery rib

1½ cups walnut milk

celery leaves

....

½ cup tamarillo flesh

1 apple

½ avocado

½ to 1 teaspoon ground cinnamon

1½ cups almond milk

greens

....

1 cup papaya

1 banana

1 whole lemon

1½ cups water

parsley

....

4 oranges and/or tangelos, peeled

1 to 2 tablespoons chia seeds

1 cup fennel juice

fennel tops

---

2 bananas

1 large pear

1 teaspoon Instant Chai Spice Mix (page 230)

1 inch fresh ginger

1½ cups almond milk

greens

---

1 cup tamarillo flesh

¼ cup raisins, soaked in water overnight

1 teaspoon vanilla extract

1½ cups almond milk

greens

---

1 cup pineapple with core

1 banana

1½ cups water

cilantro or mint

1½ cups pineapple with core

water of 1 young coconut

fennel tops

---

2 bananas

1 kiwifruit

1 tangelo

1½ cups water

cilantro

1 cup pineapple with core

½ grapefruit

½ avocado

1½ cups water

greens

½ cup young coconut flesh

juice from 1 large or 2 small pomegranates*

2 cups walnut milk or 2 cups water and 2 tablespoons walnut oil

greens

* To juice pomegranates, peel and blend whole, then strain
  through a nut milk bag or cheesecloth.

---

1 whole lemon

2 lemons, peeled

2 limes, peeled

1 inch fresh ginger

1½ cups orange juice

greens

sweetener, as needed

---

1 large pink grapefruit, peeled

1 banana

½ avocado

1½ cups orange juice

greens

Featured Recipe

Lucy Stegley (www.raweventsaustralia.com), aka SmoothieGirl, is a huge fan of raw food and smoothies. Of all the nutrition tricks, trends, and trials she's tried in her search for better health, nothing has been more life-changing and delicious than discovering and incorporating raw fruit and raw green smoothies into her diet. Here are two of her favorite winter green smoothies.

GREEN-A-COLADA

>1 cup frozen pineapple pieces
>
>1 large ripe banana
>
>1½ cups filtered or spring water or the water of 1 young Thai coconut
>
>handful of spinach
>
>5 mint leaves or pineapple sage leaves
>
>juice of ½ lime
>
>1 pitted date, pitted (optional for added sweetness)
>
>1 vanilla bean*

*In high-powered blenders, simply chop the vanilla bean in half and blend it with the smoothie. In less-powerful blenders, grind the bean separately, then blend it into the smoothie.

SPICED PEAR AND GINGER GREEN SMOOTHIE

>2 pears
>
>1 inch fresh ginger
>
>seeds of 2 cardamom pods, ground
>
>½ teaspoon ground nutmeg
>
>½ teaspoon ground cinnamon
>
>2 cups cashew milk
>
>greens

Antioxidants

Antioxidants, which exist in plants and algae, are the ideal army to fight free radicals. It is believed that free radical damage can accelerate the progression of cancer, cardiovascular disease, rheumatoid arthritis, chronic fatigue, and age-related diseases. Examples of antioxidant substances are Vitamins A, C, and E, the mineral selenium, co-enzyme Q10, glutathione, flavonoids, polyphenols, and pigments like chlorophyll and carotenoids that color plants. Oxygen Radical Absorbance Capacity (ORAC) is a standardized measurement of a food's total antioxidant power, its ability to neutralize free radicals. See page TK for more information of antioxidants and the ORAC scale.

These fruit are rich in antioxidants:

- acai berries
- apples
- blueberries
- cranberries
- figs
- goji berries
- maqui berries
- oranges
- pomegranates
- plums
- prunes
- raisins
- raspberries
- red grapes
- strawberries

In particular, goji berries, which are usually purchased dried, have a high ORAC score of around 24,000. Acai berries and maqui berries are antioxidant powerhouses: Amazonian acai can have an ORAC score between 50,000 and 101,000, depending on the quality, while Patagonian maqui can be over 300,000! These berries can usually be found in antioxidant formulas that are liquids or freeze-dried powders. Powders are better, as they don't contain preservatives. ORAC scores vary according to the quality of the produce.

Excellent antioxidant greens include:

- alfalfa sprouts
- basil
- beet stems and leaves
- cilantro
- kale
- mint
- parsley
- red leaf lettuces
- spinach

You can also boost your green smoothie's antioxidant power with spices like ground cinnamon, ginger, and cloves. Raw cacao has a very high ORAC score of 95,000 to 98,000, and pecans, hazelnuts, and walnuts have the highest ORAC scores of all nuts. Chia seeds more than double their antioxidant value when they're soaked in water.

You'll get a high dose of antioxidants from micro-algae like spirulina, chlorella, AFA, and marine phytoplankton, and supplements like Berry Radical Antioxidant Superfood, which has an ORAC score of 117,500.

Antioxidant-Boosting Recipes

Superfood powders and micro-algae can be added to any smoothie for extra antioxidant power. Because antioxidants are frequently bitter, smoothie recipes may need extra sweetener; choose which one at your discretion and add as needed.

1 to 2 bananas

½ cup fresh berries, any variety

¼ cup goji berries, soaked

1½ cups water

greens

---

4 fresh figs

1 cup red grapes

4 walnut halves

1½ cups water

spinach

small handful of basil leaves

---

2 apples

I banana

½ teaspoon ground cinnamon

2 tablespoons acai or maqui berry powder

1 teaspoon vanilla extract

kale

---

1 cup pitted cherries

2 oranges, peeled

2 tablespoons hemp seeds

juice of 2 oranges

greens

I cup unhulled strawberries

handful of goji berries

flesh and water of 1 young coconut

handful of mint

¼ cup diced beets

1 apple

1 orange

1 tablespoon raw cacao

1½ cups pecan or walnut milk

greens

juice of 1 large or 2 small pomegranates*

2 oranges

½ teaspoon ground cinnamon

4 walnut halves

large handful of parsley

*To juice pomegranates, peel and blend whole, then strain
 through a nut milk bag or cheesecloth.

2 pears

1 inch fresh ginger

1 teaspoon Instant Chai Spice Mix (page 230)

1 to 2 tablespoons raw cacao powder (optional)

1½ cups hazelnut milk

spinach

2 bananas

1 cup blueberries

2 tablespoons raw cacao powder

1 teaspoon vanilla extract

handful of mint

Featured Recipe

Scott Fry is the director of Loving Earth (www.lovingearth.net), a Melbourne-based company dedicated to sourcing the highest quality organic and wild-harvested functional foods from around the world. During midmorning at Loving Earth headquarters, you can usually hear their blender whirling up a green smoothie in the staff kitchen. Richard, one of the production managers, usually appears with a mug in hand waiting expectantly for Scott to finish making a blender full of this green smoothie bursting with antioxidant power:

  4 cups or handfuls curly kale leaf

  4 cups filtered water

  juice of 6 oranges

  4 bananas

  2 tablespoons E3Live AFA Powder

  2 tablespoons yacon syrup

  1 tablespoon Gubinge Powder (or other food-based, high-vitamin C powder)

  1 tablespoon maqui berry powder

  1 tablespoon melted coconut oil or hemp seed oil

Says Scott:

  The base of water, kale, orange juice, and bananas can be mixed with whatever else you want, or you can have it just straight up and simple. It is so simple, yet delicious. We add the full spectrum of superfoods and a little yacon syrup to sweeten it and keep your probiotics humming along. Enjoy, and feel the massive health benefits!

  1 cup plums

  ⅛ teaspoon ground cloves

  zest of ½ orange

  1 orange, peeled

  1½ cups walnut milk

  1 teaspoon vanilla extract

  greens

1 cup cranberries

2 cups frozen orange segments

½ teaspoon ground cinnamon

½ cup water

greens

Bones and Joints

Bone health is very complex, and managing it involves a balance of minerals, vitamins, enzymes, and hormones, not to mention weight-bearing exercise! Our bones are made up primarily of calcium, and modern medicine would lead you to believe that all you need for bone health is calcium and vitamin D. However, bone density is determined by many factors. For healthy, strong bones we need hormone balance, a broad spectrum of vitamins and minerals, and a mostly alkaline-forming, rather than acid-forming, diet.

An acid-forming lifestyle contains a lot of sugar, alcohol, stress, highly processed grains, meat, and junk food. Acid formation in the blood is balanced by alkaline minerals such as calcium and magnesium. So the issue of poor bone density is not logically managed by throwing calcium tablets into the system, but rather by asking why the calcium has been depleted. Reducing the need for supplemental calcium by eating an alkaline-forming diet makes more sense, as does supplying the body with organic minerals from plants, not from crushed up tablets that are poorly utilized by the body.

Green smoothies are naturally alkaline forming, and vitamin and mineral rich. Vitamins and key and trace minerals for bone health such as vitamin C, magnesium, and manganese can be boosted by:

- almonds
- cacao
- cashews
- chia seeds
- pineapple
- pumpkinseeds
- sunflower seeds

And drink your smoothie in the sun each day for the best source of vitamin D!

Healthy bones are a matrix of minerals that create a hard skeleton. Joints are where the two hard, bony ends meet. Most joints in the body are synovial joints like fingers, hips, and knees. This means they are enclosed in a soft tissue capsule that contains a small amount of fluid to lubricate and nourish the joint surfaces. These joints are prone to degeneration and inflammation if stressed by suboptimal nutrition or external stress such as an injury.

Joint-friendly green smoothie ingredients are anti-inflammatory by nature, including:

- avocados (for vitamin E)
- berries high in anti-oxidants (see page 130) and with rich pigments
- Brazil nuts (for selenium)
- fruits rich in vitamin C
- kale
- micro-algae
- spinach
- sunflower oil and seeds (organic)

Omega-3 oils from chia seeds, flax seeds, walnuts, and micro-algae convert to anti-inflammatory prostaglandins. Omega-6

GLA in spirulina, borage, and hemp seeds are naturally anti-inflammatory, as are alfalfa, aloe vera, ginger, and MSM powder.

Bone- and Joint-Friendly Recipes

Algae such as AFA and spirulina, MSM, and oils such as flax seed and walnut can be added to any smoothie for extra bone and joint health. Go easy on the MSM powder as the flavor can be unpleasant in quantities of more than 2 teaspoons:

1 banana

1 cup berries, any variety

2 tablespoons hemp seeds

1½ cups water

greens

2 cups sweet citrus segments

½ avocado

2 teaspoons spirulina powder

1 cup water

greens

2 large ripe pears

1 inch fresh ginger

1½ cups seed milk

greens

flesh of 3 lemons

zest of 1 lemon

1 tablespoons MSM powder

1½ cups orange juice

parsley

sweetener of choice, as needed

2 bananas

2 tablespoons raw cacao

1 tablespoon chia seeds

1½ cups Brazil nut milk

greens

....

2 frozen bananas

I cup unhulled strawberries

AFA algae

spinach

Featured Recipe

Nutritionist **Cyndi O'Meara** (www.changinghabits.com.au) is the author of the best-selling book *Changing Habits Changing Lives*. Cyndi is not your stereotypical nutritionist—she disagrees with low-fat, low-calorie diets and believes chocolate can be good for you! Cyndi is a huge fan of green smoothies and devotes a section to the humble drink in her fantastic diabetes report, available on her website www.changinghabits.com.au.

This green smoothie recipe from Cyndi is bursting with bone- and joint-friendly ingredients. Serves 2.

CYNDI'S PURPLE CHOC GREEN SMOOTHIE

    1 large ripe banana

    3 to 4 cups spinach

    3 fresh dates, pitted

    1 cup frozen blueberries

    1 tablespoon raw cacao powder

    5 cashews

    1 teaspoon Changing Habits Supreme Green Blend

    1 teaspoon Changing Habits Organic Colloidal Minerals

    1 teaspoon Changing Habits Rapadura Sugar

    pinch of Changing Habits Seaweed Salt

    5 ice cubes

    1½ cups water

1 cup pineapple with core

1 banana

inner leaf gel from 4 inches aloe vera

mint

alfalfa sprouts

---

2 oranges, peeled

1 banana

1½ cups pecan or walnut milk

greens

---

1 orange, peeled

1 mango

1 inch fresh ginger

1 tablespoon chia seeds

1½ cups water

Bowel

"Death begins in the colon."
—*Nobel Laureate Ilya Mechnikov*

A healthy bowel needs an ideal balance of good and bad bacteria—about 80 percent good and 20 percent bad, which is frequently the opposite in an unhealthy gut—and the bowel's contents need to move with an adequate supply of fiber.

Green smoothies are fiber rich by nature because of the greens and fruit content. The greener the smoothie, the more fiber it will contain. Extra fiber-rich additions can include chia seeds, beets, and oats. Soluble fiber–rich fruits are most ideal and include:

- apples
- bananas
- blueberries
- citrus (peeled)
- kiwifruit

- mangoes
- pears
- plums
- strawberries

Some people, however, cannot handle a fiber-rich diet and are prone to diarrhea if they consume too much fiber for their digestive tract. A friend of mine has a "fussy tummy" like this, and she wishes she could eat more greens and fruit. Our challenge has been to create lower fiber green smoothies for her and we have succeeded. (See "Fussy About Fruit" on page 207 for more details.)

Bacterial imbalance (or dysbiosis) is a common problem affecting the bowel. It can lead to food sensitivities, carbohydrate cravings, fatigue, irritable bowel symptoms, acid reflux, poor sleep, painful joints, gum disease, frequent colds and flu, acne, eczema, hormone imbalance, and yeast problems like candida and athlete's foot. So it certainly seems that getting the gut working well gets just about everything else working well!

If you do not eat probiotic-rich, fermented foods very regularly, probiotic supplements should ideally be taken daily or multiple times daily in times of stress or illness. My preferred bacterial supplement is In-Liven Fermented Probiotic Superfood (see page 95), which also contains spirulina and other green foods. Spirulina works in harmony with lactobacillus bacteria by aiding its reproductive ability in the gut. Probiotics ultimately assist almost every function in the human body, and in the stomach they will help to calm an irritated bowel prone to diarrhea, help a constipated bowel to get moving, and help conquer candida overgrowth.

For digestive systems prone to candida or inflammation, excellent additions to green smoothies include coconut, chia seeds, aloe vera, noni, and slippery elm powder. Cooled herbal teas can be used instead of water and include those made from horsetail, pau d'arco, marshmallow, and lemon myrtle. For people choosing a fruit- and sugar-free diet for strict candida management, check out "Savory Smoothies" on page 220.

High-Fiber Recipes to Really Get Things Moving!

Be as generous as possible with greens. Chia can be added to any smoothie for extra fiber, and probiotics are recommended to be added to smoothies daily.

⅛ cup oat groats, soaked overnight, drained, and rinsed

2 bananas

1½ cups water

greens

¼ cup diced beets

2 large pears

1½ cups nut milk

greens

---

1 mango

2 oranges, peeled, leaving some pith

1 cup water

greens

---

6 prunes

2 bananas

1 pear

1½ cups water

greens

---

1 cup unhulled strawberries

2 kiwifruit with skin

2 tablespoons chia seeds

1 cup water

greens

1 pear

1 banana

1 cup blueberries

1 cup water

greens

Green Smoothies High in Soluble Fiber

Here are some recipes to help soothe sensitive digestive systems not prone to diarrhea.

Chia can be added to all smoothies for extra soluble fiber, as can probiotics and also slippery elm powder. Herbs such as mint, basil, cilantro, and parsley can be used for their stomach-soothing properties. For stomachs prone to diarrhea, try the green smoothie recipes promoting good bowel health on page 141.

1 banana

1 cup red papaya

1½ cups water

greens

2 bananas

1 very ripe pear

1½ cups water

mint

1 very ripe mango

inner leaf gel of 4 inches aloe vera

1½ cups cooled marshmallow tea

greens

1 banana

2 very ripe pears

2 tablespoons chia seeds

1½ cups cooled horsetail tea

greens

---

2 oranges, peeled

1 banana

1½ cups cooled lemon myrtle tea

greens

---

1 cup red papaya

½ cup young coconut flesh

honey

1½ cups cooled pau d'arco tea

greens

Cardiovascular Health

There are many complicated chemical reactions in our bodies, and if certain nutrients are missing, then processes can get stuck. In some of these "stuck" situations, an amino acid called homocysteine can rise to dangerous levels. High levels of homocysteine are known to be associated with cardiovascular diseases like heart attack and stroke, as well as neural tube defects, osteoporosis, Alzheimer's disease, cancer, liver disease, depression, and peripheral neuropathy. Homocysteine in high amounts can damage artery walls, leading to inflammation and atherosclerosis.

High homocysteine levels are a more reliable predictor of cardiovascular disease than high cholesterol levels are, so for good cardiovascular health, we want our diets to discourage the rise of homocysteine. A diet very high in animal products will supply a lot of the amino acid methionine, which turns into homocysteine.

In addition to a low-toxic, plant-based diet, specific nutrients are required to ensure the beneficial chain of chemical reactions occurs within our cells. These nutrients include vitamins B2, B6, and B12, folic acid, magnesium, and zinc. Fruits and greens supply many nutrients required for keeping homocysteine levels down, such as antioxidants, vitamin C, vitamin E, and minerals, which are staple ingredients in green smoothies. An alkaline diet rich in blended greens and probiotics should result in adequate B12 levels. It's wise to have B12 tested, especially for strict vegans; however, meat eaters can be deficient, too, if their ability to absorb it is a problem.

Homocysteine lacks a "methyl" group, so anything that can donate a methyl group is very helpful, for example the methylcobalamin form of vitamin B12, the methyl group from MSM (methylsulfonylmethane), and the methyl group in TMG (trimethylglycine). Here are some good homocysteine-lowering foods:

- beets
- eggs
- goji berries
- nuts
- seeds
- soy lecithin
- sunflower oil (organic, cold-pressed)

TMG, also known as betaine, is found in raw foods, particularly in beets and goji berries. Betain pigments in beets also help with glutathione function, so beets, including the stems and leaves, are excellent for cardiovascular health. Choline is needed to make TMG in the body, and exists in soy lecithin, sunflower oil (use only organic, cold-pressed), and most nuts, including peanuts, and seeds, as well as eggs.

High homocysteine also tends to coincide with low levels of glutathione, one of the most important liver-detoxifying antioxidants. Other glutathione-boosting foods suitable for green smoothies include:

- avocados
- Brazil nuts
- cabbage
- cardamom
- chia seeds
- cinnamon
- flax seeds
- kale
- micro-algae
- peaches
- sunflower seeds
- walnuts
- watermelon

Also important for cardiovascular health is vitamin K, a very important blood-clotting agent. Greens rich in vitamin K are:

- chard
- collards
- kale
- parsley
- spinach

Recipes to Optimize Cardiovascular Health

3 bananas

½ teaspoon ground cinnamon

¼ teaspoon ground cardamom

1½ cups Brazil nut milk

bok choy

½ cup blueberries

¼ cup goji berries, soaked

flesh and water of 1 young Thai coconut

beet greens with stems

sweetener, as needed

2 peaches

1 banana

2 teaspoons spirulina or AFA algae

2 tablespoons organic sunflower oil

2 cups water

kale

4 cups watermelon

4 tablespoons chia seeds

mint

greens

1 apple

¼ cup diced beets

½ small avocado

1 tablespoon raw cacao powder

1 cup ice cubes

1 cup apple juice

beet greens and stems

1 banana

2 pears

1 teaspoon vanilla extract

1½ cups sunflower seed milk

greens

2 bananas

4 dried figs, soaked in water overnight

2 tablespoons soy lecithin or organic sunflower oil

1½ cups water

greens

1 cup grapes (any variety)

2 oranges, peeled

2 tablespoons chia seeds

2 tablespoons walnut oil

1 cup water

greens

---

2 bananas

2 tablespoons peanut butter

2 cups water or nut milk

greens

---

2 peaches

1 cup berries

1½ cups water

¼ avocado

greens

Cellular Health

Our entire body is made up of cells, so our cellular health is pretty important! It's no understatement to say that we need a bit of everything to keep our cells working in tip-top shape. What are cells? They are microscopic and spherical, and each cell is like a factory that has a power source (mitochondria), workers (ribosomes), a boss (DNA in the nucleus), security (cell walls), and logistics (coordination of transport in and out of the cell). The function of a cell is complex and relies on everyone doing their job and external factors being ideal. If anything upsets the cell's process, bad things can happen.

The way our bodies grow and heal is reliant on healthy cells dividing into more identical healthy cells. Unhealthy cells can explode, shrink, or mutate. Mutated cells, if allowed to divide over and over, can cause cancerous tumors. When cells are healthy and the body's immune system is strong, cell mutations are minimal and the body quickly identifies and kills them off before they have a chance to divide.

To try and keep our cells living healthily and keeping mutations at bay, we need to ensure we are well hydrated; we need to avoid toxins, eat plenty of antioxidant-rich foods, and eat mineral-rich foods, in particular those containing selenium, manganese, magnesium, and zinc. We need to keep our homocysteine levels down (see "Cardiovascular Health" on page 146), ensure we consume all eight essential amino acids, eat essential fats, supplement with probiotics, and eat enzyme- and vitamin-rich food.

Fruits, greens, and water present in green smoothies will supply us with hydration, antioxidants, minerals, enzymes, amino acids, and vitamins.

Raw honey is also a fantastic source of enzymes. Pineapple is the richest source of manganese, which is necessary for many enzyme reactions in the body. Manganese is also present in leafy greens, maple syrup, grapes, red berries, and bananas. Sulforaphane, an organic sulfur-bearing compound, is formed when cruciferous vegetables such as kale are chopped, chewed, or blended. Sulforaphane has been shown in experimental studies to have anti-cancer, anti-microbial, and anti-diabetic properties.

A variety of different leafy greens, herbs, microgreens, sprouts, and seeds will ensure we receive all essential amino acids to build proteins for enzymes, hormones, and muscle tissue. Some fantastic sources include:

- Brazil nuts
- chia seeds
- flax seeds
- oats
- pumpkinseeds
- sesame seeds
- spinach
- sunflower seeds

Seeds like chia, sesame, sunflower, and pumpkin provide us with vitamin E, magnesium, zinc, amino acids, and omega-3 and -6 fats. Just one or two Brazil nuts per day is considered sufficient to supply us with enough of the antioxidant mineral selenium, which is also present in spinach, oats, and sunflower seeds.

Chia seed and flax seed are the highest plant sources of omega-3 essential fats. Because chia is antioxidant rich, it is more stable and does not go rapidly rancid like flax does. Chia is also more digestible, as it fully softens with soaking and does not have any taste, unlike flax, which can have a strong, bitter, nutty flavor when ground or as oil, and it is not very conducive to sweet green smoothies.

Specific homocysteine-lowering green smoothie additions include:

- avocado
- apricots (dried)
- bananas
- beets
- dates
- figs
- oranges
- soy lecithin
- sunflower oil (organic)
- walnuts

Probiotics are abundant in fermented foods, which are generally not green smoothie friendly. While some people like to add kefir (fermented milk) to their smoothies for a probiotic boost, I prefer to add lactobacillus probiotics to keep my daily smoothie plant based.

Cellular Health–Boosting Recipes

2 to 3 bananas

1 tablespoon chia seeds

maple syrup, as needed

1½ cups Brazil nut milk

greens

1 cup pineapple with core

1 orange, peeled

2 tablespoons chia seeds

1½ cups water

cilantro and/or mint

¼ cup diced beets

1 cup raspberries

2 Medjool dates

1 cup ice cubes

1 cup sesame milk

1 tablespoon walnut oil

greens

⅛ cup oat groats, soaked overnight, drained, and rinsed

1 banana

2 fresh or soaked dried figs

1½ cups water

greens

1 cup unhulled strawberries

zest of ½ lemon

½ avocado

1½ cups sunflower seed or pumpkinseed milk

greens

2 oranges, peeled

¼ cup dried apricots, soaked overnight

1 tablespoon soy lecithin or organic sunflower oil

1½ cups water

greens

Featured Recipe

Narelle Chenery is the founder and creative director of research and development for Miessence (www.miessence.com), the world's first extensive range of internationally certified organic skin, hair, body, cosmetic, oral, and nutritional products. Narelle is a huge fan of green smoothies, and this is her version loaded with cellular health–boosting ingredients! Serves 2.

> juice and flesh of 1 baby green coconut
>
> ½ cup of fruit of the season (papaya, mango, peaches, pears, berries)
>
> 1 banana
>
> handful of goji berries
>
> 1 teaspoon bee pollen
>
> 1 teaspoon maca root powder
>
> 2 teaspoons In-Liven Fermented Probiotic Superfood
>
> 2 teaspoons Berry Radical Antioxidant Superfood
>
> 2 teaspoons Deep Green Alkaliser
>
> 2 tablespoons soaked chia seeds
>
> big handful of spinach or other leafy greens
>
> 1 tablespoon flax oil, evening primrose oil, hemp oil, or a good EFA (essential fatty acid) blend
>
> 4 tablespoons hemp protein or protein powder of choice

Says Narelle:

This morning smoothie is a meal that keeps us going until lunchtime. It's got everything you need in it. Loads of phytonutrition! Greens, antioxidants, probiotics, and the macronutrients (protein, oils, and fiber). Plus it's delicious.

> 2 to 3 bananas
>
> 2 tablespoons raw cacao
>
> 1½ cups sunflower seed or pumpkinseed milk
>
> mint

1 cup red grapes

4 dried figs, soaked overnight

1½ cups water

1 tablespoon walnut oil

greens

----

2 cups pineapple with core

flesh and water of 1 young coconut

greens

----

2 lemons, whole or peeled and pith removed

2 oranges, peeled

2 mandarin oranges, peeled

½ cup ice cubes

1 cup water

kale

sweetener, as needed

----

2 bananas

1 lemon, peeled

2 tablespoons raw wild honey

1 tablespoon bee pollen

1½ cups water or nut milk

greens

Good Blood Sugar

As discussed in "Can Green Smoothies Help with Weight Loss?" (page 68), factors that influence steady blood sugar are fiber-dense foods, particularly those containing soluble fiber; combining protein and carbohydrates; low–glycemic load (GL) carbohydrates; minerals chromium, magnesium, and zinc; vitamin C; cinnamon; cilantro; and the avoidance of stimulants such as caffeine and stress.

Fruits high in soluble fiber include:

- apples
- bananas
- blueberries
- citrus (whole, peeled)
- kiwifruit
- mangoes
- plums
- pears
- strawberries

Most of these fruits also contain vitamin C.

Greens are abundant in insoluble fiber, are mineral and protein rich, and some contain good amounts of vitamin C, such as:

- beet greens
- kale
- parsley

Protein and minerals can be boosted in green smoothies by the addition of chia seeds, hemp seeds, spirulina, soaked raw nuts and seeds, and nut or seed milks. For those wishing to boost protein further, Sunwarrior Protein Powder is made from fermented brown rice and is a raw, vegan alternative to using whey protein powders.

People who are significantly hypoglycemic who are not opposed to using animal products in their smoothies may find it beneficial to add probiotic yogurt, kefir, or eggs. See the "Fussy About Fruit" on page 207 for recipes.

Recipes for Blood-Sugar Maintenance

Extra protein in the form of spirulina or whey/rice protein powder can be added to your daily smoothie as desired, as can cinnamon or chia seeds. Water can be substituted for any of the nut or seed milks; however, if you do use water, add another source of minerals and protein, such as chia seeds.

> 1 small banana
>
> 1 apple
>
> 1 pear
>
> 1½ cups almond milk
>
> 1 teaspoon ground cinnamon
>
> greens

> 1 pear
>
> 2 cups of mandarin orange, peeled
>
> 2 to 3 tablespoons hemp seeds
>
> 1 cup water
>
> greens

1 small banana

1 cup blueberries

2 tablespoons chia seeds

1½ cups water

greens

½ mango

1 cup unhulled strawberries

1½ cups cashew milk

greens

½ cup plums

zest of ½ orange

2 oranges, peeled

1 teaspoon cinnamon

2 to 3 tablespoons hemp seeds

greens

1 small banana

I kiwifruit (skin optional)

1 cup unhulled strawberries

1½ cups almond milk

2 tablespoons chia seeds

greens

½ mango

2 cups sweet citrus segments

zest ½ lemon

2 tablespoons sunflower seeds, preferably soaked

1½ cups water

greens

2 pears

1 orange, peeled

1 to 2 teaspoons Instant Chai Spice Mix (page 230)

1½ cups nut milk or water

greens

2 cups mandarin oranges, peeled

2 plums

1½ cups pumpkinseed milk

greens

1 lemon, quartered (remove some seeds if there are lots)

3 tablespoons chia seeds

1 cup ice cubes

2 cups orange juice

cilantro

Weight Loss

As previously discussed, adding green smoothies to regular diets and to raw food diets frequently results in assistance with weight control, and it's easy to see why—green smoothies check all the boxes regarding blood sugar control and satiation. Green smoothies:

- Contain fiber
- Are usually low glycemic load (GL), unless loaded with bananas and sweeteners
- Contain protein and carbohydrates
- Are highly nutritious
- Supply good-quality fuel for cells without side effects
- Are alkaline and therefore calming (nonstressful) to the body
- If made from organic food sources are more likely to supply trace minerals low or absent in conventional produce

If the addition of green smoothies does not result in weight loss, then aiming for low-GL smoothies and a low-GL diet overall is recommended (see page TK). The Holford Diet, as described by Patrick Holford, a UK-based nutritionist, proposes eating no more than 40 GL points daily (10 per meal and two

5 GL snacks or drinks), and eating carbohydrates with protein. Because GL takes the concept of GI a step further by taking into account the portion of food, this means, for example, that a green smoothie should not contain more than half a banana per serving, as one banana has a GL of 12. The same smoothie should also not contain any other high-GL fruits like mangoes, grapes, or extra sweeteners like honey or dates.

The Holford Diet is also plant based, rich in essential fats, and places an emphasis on nutrient-rich whole foods and the consumption of raw and minimally cooked fruit and vegetables. Cyndi O'Meara, a nutritionist from Australia, proposes a similar eating plan without the counting of points. Her emphasis is on eating real, unprocessed foods that are also rich in plant foods, raw foods, and essential fats and proteins. Neither eating plan is vegetarian nor raw, unlike the diets that green smoothie drinkers are frequently associated with; however, green smoothies can benefit any diet as it will move consumers toward a more nutritious way of eating.

Recipes to Aid Weight Loss

All of these recipes are less than 20 GL for 1 liter/1 quart of smoothie, which is enough for a serving each for two people, or for two separate meals in a day of 10 GL or less each. The GL of each ingredient is listed in parenthesis. The total GL for the smoothie is given at the end. For a complete list of GL for common foods, visit www.gl.patrickholford.interactiveprofiling. com, where you can also build a GL-appropriate menu. www .nutritiondata.com also details the GLs of the many foods on their site.

2 cups mixed berries (2)

2 pears (10)

1½ cups water or nut milk (0)

greens (1)

Total 13

---

1 banana (12)

1 cup blueberries (2)

1½ cups water or nut milk (0)

greens (1)

Total 15

½ cantaloupe (10)

1 cup unhulled strawberries (5)

1 cup water (0)

greens (1)

Total 16

---

1 cup pitted cherries (5)

2 oranges (10)

1½ cups water or nut milk (0)

greens (1)

Total 16

---

3 peaches (15)

½ cup raspberries (1)

1 teaspoon vanilla extract (0)

1½ cups water (0)

greens (1)

Total 17

1 orange (5)

½ mango (10)

1 lime, peeled (1)

1½ cups water (0)

greens (1)

stevia, as needed (0)

Total 17

4 apricots (5)

1 banana (12)

1 teaspoon vanilla extract (0)

½ to 1 teaspoon ground cinnamon (0)

1½ cups water or nut milk (0)

greens (1)

Total 18

1 banana (12)

1 pear (5)

¼ cup hemp seeds (0)

1½ cups water (0)

greens (1)

Total 18

2 cups watermelon (17)

1 cup water (0)

greens and mint (1)

Total 18

1 cup pineapple with core (10)

1 small grapefruit, peeled (5)

flesh and 1 cup water from a young coconut (3)

greens (1)

Total 19

Featured Recipe

Jemma Gawned, creator and director of Naked Treaties Rawganics (www .nakedtreaties.com.au), has been a raw food and green smoothie advocate since 2006. Jemma loves her green smoothies really green, not too thick, and very cleansing. Jemma's really, really green smoothie is also low GL:

water of 1 young coconut
3 or 4 massive handfuls of greens
1 banana or ½ mango
1 cup raspberries or strawberries
flesh of 1 passion fruit

Happy Hormones

There are many types of hormones in the body, including insulin for blood sugar control, serotonin for mood, and thyroxine for the thyroid. The hormones we'll talk about here are the sex hormones, such as progesterone, estrogen, and testosterone. Progesterone and estrogen are considered the female hormones and testosterone the male; however, all three are present in males and females, just in different amounts.

When hormones are imbalanced, the estrogen to testosterone/progesterone ratio is generally too high. Hence a very important part of hormone health is to avoid becoming estrogen dominant. Xeno-estrogens, or bad estrogens, mimic real estrogen and come from plastics, toxic fumes, pesticides, and chemicals used in personal care and cosmetics. When xeno-estrogens are added to naturally occurring estrogens in the body, the total amount becomes dominant to the androgen group of hormones (progesterone, testosterone, and DHEA). Symptoms of estrogen dominance can include infertility, bad menopausal symptoms, PMS, polycystic ovaries, breast cancer, mood swings, osteoporosis, acne, migraines, and prostate cancer.

Avoiding xeno-estrogens exposure is vital: reduce or eliminate the use of plastic containers for storage and drinking; eat organic food; and use personal care products and cosmetics that are free of synthetic chemicals. There are also substances that can help remove these bad estrogens from the body, including lemon and lime peel, apples, pears, berries, cruciferous vegetables, and iodine-rich foods such as seaweed.

Bad estrogens and homocysteine (see "Cardiovascular Health" on page 146) both lack a methyl group. Foods that help to decrease homocysteine by donating a methyl group also help with the removal of bad estrogens. Many of these foods include the compound betaine, which is found in beets, spinach and goji berries, avocado, MSM, and lots of leafy greens.

In addition to a whole-food, plant-based diet, hormone health can be boosted by adequate intake of essential fats, vitamins B3 and B6, and the minerals magnesium and zinc.

Vitamin B3 is not abundant in green smoothie–friendly ingredients, but it can be found in excellent amounts in cremini and shiitake mushrooms, and in lesser amounts in:

- cantaloupe
- chard
- collard greens
- fennel
- mustard greens
- raspberries
- romaine lettuce
- tomatoes
- turnip greens

Vitamin B6 can be found in:

- bananas
- bell peppers
- celery
- greens
- watermelon

Magnesium and zinc can be found in:

- cacao
- chia seeds
- leafy greens

- pumpkinseeds
- sunflower seeds

Excellent fat sources are coconut, chia seed, flax seed, and hemp seed. The omega-6 oil GLA is very hormone friendly and can be found in borage, spirulina, and evening primrose.

Herbs such as agnus castus (vitex), dong quai (angelica), black cohosh, and St. John's wort are often used for hormone imbalance issues, and cooled tea made from these herbs can be used as a base for a green smoothie. Such herbs are ideally used on the professional advice of a naturopath or herbalist.

Maca is a superfood root crop from the time of the ancient Incas. It contains many vitamins, minerals, enzymes, and unique alkaloids that work as an adaptogen to hormones, meaning they can help to balance whatever hormone is out of balance, as opposed to influencing just a single hormone (for example, vitex primarily only influences progesterone. Maca has a strong flavor, so I recommend using a small amount in a green smoothie and drinking it immediately, as the maca has a tendency to developing an unpleasant radishlike flavor if left to sit.

In Eastern medicine, decreased *jing* energy can be part of hormone issues such as infertility; both maca and parsley are good for increasing *jing*. Cacao and bee pollen are also hormone-friendly foods, as are passion flower, chamomile, fennel, anise, and resveratrol in grapes.

Hormone-Friendly Recipes

Prioritize the use of the following greens: cruciferous greens such as kale, collards, and bok choy, spinach, romaine, turnip greens, beet greens, borage leaves and flowers, celery tops, anise and fennel tops, and parsley.

Add micro-algae, particularly spirulina, to any or all recipes.

Consider using cooled teas as liquids, including passion flower, chamomile, fennel, and anise.

2 to 3 bananas
½ cup goji berries (preferably soaked)
1½ cups water or seed milk
greens

3 cups watermelon (include the seeds)
1 whole lime, quartered
1 inch fresh ginger
greens

3 to 4 bananas
1 tablespoon maca
1 tablespoon bee pollen
1½ cups water or nut/seed milk
greens

flesh and water of 1 Thai coconut
juice and peel of 1 lime
1 cup raspberries
greens

2 cups cantaloupe

½ cup raspberries

1 cup water

greens

2 bananas

flesh and peel of 1 large lemon

2 teaspoon MSM powder

½ avocado

1½ cups water

parsley

2 cups red grapes

peel of 1 lime

3 tablespoons chia seeds

1½ cups nut/seed milk

greens

¼ cup diced beet

2 apples

2 cups nut/seed milk

greens

1 cup tomatoes

1 medium red pepper, seeded

1 cup celery tops

peel of 1 lemon

1 teaspoon dulse flakes

1 cup of ice

3 frozen bananas

2 tablespoons raw cacao

1 tablespoon maca

2 servings medicinal mushroom powder or liquid

1½ cups water

greens

---

3 pears

1½ cups water

¼ cup hemp seeds

2 teaspoons Instant Chai Spice Mix (page 230)

Longevity

The secret to longevity is no magic pill or potion, nor is there one single diet that appears to be the best. All the long-lived populations in the world could not have more varied diets. The key factor that links them all together is the absence of synthetic chemicals and processed food. That is those people ate "real food" and had lifestyles devoid of modern-day stressors.

We can't exactly all give up our lives and move to wild or remote places like the populations that are known for longevity, like the Hunzas, Vilcabambans, or Okinawins. But it's good to know what we can do in our lives now. The key factors appear to be keeping homocysteine low (see "Cardiovascular Health" on page 146), and eating a diet rich in antioxidants, leafy greens, and B vitamins.

The following fruits are excellent for longevity:

- apples
- avocados
- berries (especially acai, goji, and maqui)
- figs
- oranges
- peaches
- pomegranates
- plums
- prunes
- raisins
- red grapes
- watermelon

Greens ideal for longevity include:

- basil and other herbs
- beet greens and stems
- chard
- cilantro
- collards
- kale
- microgreens
- mint
- parsley
- purslane
- red leaf lettuces
- spinach
- sprouts

The following ingredients suit green smoothies for longevity:

- cacao
- cardamom
- chia seeds
- cinnamon
- cloves
- ginger
- micro-algae
- nuts (including peanuts)
- sunflower seeds and oil

Recent research also points to what determines our lifespan. At birth we have 10,000 base pairs of telomeres on the DNA in our cells. By death we have around 5,000. Hence we lose 50 base pairs about once a year. TA65 is a substance that is called a telomerase activator, which is supposed to add base back on to our telomeres. Exciting stuff! Both purslane and astragalus root contain TA65, and most TA65 supplements are made from astragalus root.

Antiaging Recipes to Start Turning Back the Clock!

Superfood powders and micro-algae can be added to any smoothie for extra nutrition and antioxidant power. Astragalus root preparations can also be added, or use cooled astragalus tea as the liquid.

3 bananas

2 teaspoons Instant Chai Spice Mix (page 230)

1½ cups Brazil nut milk

greens

½ cup blueberries

½ cup soaked goji berries

flesh and milk from a young Thai coconut

beet greens with stems

sweetener, to taste

----

2 peaches

1 banana

2 tablespoon organic sunflower oil

2 teaspoons spirulina or AFA algae

2 cups water

greens

----

4 cups watermelon

4 tablespoons chia seeds

1 inch fresh ginger

mint

greens

----

1 apple

¼ cup diced beet

½ small avocado

1 tablespoon raw cacao powder

1 cup apple juice

1 cup ice

beet greens and stems

2 bananas

4 dried figs, soaked overnight

2 tablespoons soy lecithin or organic sunflower oil

1½ cups water

greens

1 cup red grapes

2 oranges, peeled

2 tablespoons chia seeds

2 tablespoons walnut oil

1 cup water

greens

3 bananas

2 tablespoons peanut butter

1 to 2 tablespoons raw cacao powder

1½ cups water or nut milk

greens

1 to 2 bananas

½ cup fresh berries

¼ cup goji berries, soaked overnight (optional)

1½ cups water

greens

4 fresh figs

1 cup red grapes

4 walnut halves

1½ cups water

spinach

small handful basil leaves

2 apples

I banana

1 teaspoon ground cinnamon

2 servings acai or maqui berry

1 teaspoon vanilla extract

greens

1 cup cherries

2 oranges, peeled

2 tablespons cashews

juice of 2 oranges

greens

I pint unhulled strawberries

handful of goji berries

4 tablespoons hemp seeds

water of 1 Thai coconut

handful of mint

sweetener, as needed

1 large or 2 small pomegranates, juiced*

2 oranges

½ to 1 teaspoon ground cinnamon

4 walnut halves

large handful parsley

* To juice pomegranates, peel and blend whole, then strain
through a nut milk bag or cheesecloth.

2 pears

1 inch fresh ginger

1 teaspoon Instant Chai Spice Mix (page 230)

1 to 2 tablespoons cacao (optional)

1½ cups hazelnut milk

spinach

---

1 cup plums

⅛ teaspoon ground clove

zest of ½ orange

1 orange, peeled

1½ cups walnut milk

1 teaspoon vanilla extract

greens

---

1 cup cranberries

2 cups frozen orange segments

½ to 1 teaspoon ground cinnamon

½ cup water

greens

Beauty

Our skin is our largest organ, and there are some key factors that will help create beautiful, glowing skin!

An unhappy gut frequently manifests as a skin disorder like eczema or acne, so an alkaline diet full of greens, good-quality fiber, and probiotics is very important. Hormones can also influence skin. Essential fats, zinc, magnesium, and vitamin B6 are all necessary for hormone health and are supplied by chia seeds, sunflower seeds, pumpkinseeds, cacao, hemp seeds, bananas, dried fruits and greens, as well as hormone-friendly foods like maca, lemon peel, beets, goji berries, and avocados.

Sulfur is an important beauty mineral, so try cruciferous vegetables like kale, collards, and cabbage leaves in your green smoothies, along with MSM powder. More than a couple teaspoons of MSM can taste quite unpleasant, but it will become more pleasing over time and is masked well by lemon, which is good because vitamin C and MSM are an excellent combination for optimal nutrient absorption. Silica is another important beauty mineral and can be found in cucumbers, oats, strawberries, avocados, horsetail, comfrey, and nettle. Antioxidants are also vital for cellular health and part of our anti-aging brigade of free radical fighters. So plenty of berries, kale, alfalfa sprouts, micro-algae, and cacao are definitely in order!

In David Wolfe's book *Eating for Beauty* he includes the following as his most beautifying foods: aloe vera, arugula, burdock root, coconuts and coconut oil, cucumbers, durian, figs, hemp seeds, macadamias, nettles, olives, onions, papaya, pumpkinseeds, radishes, turmeric, and watercress.

Don't forget water! In addition to the invaluable hydration green smoothies provide, be sure to drink enough fluids, ideally around 2 quarts of good-quality water daily, and more if it is hot or you are exercising.

Beautifying Recipes

For variety, in place of water in a smoothie, try a cooled tea such as horsetail, nettle, comfrey, echinacea, chamomile, or dandelion. All smoothies can have MSM and/or micro-algae such as AFA and spirulina added on a daily basis:

1 banana
1 cup papaya
1 lemon, quartered
parsley
1½ cups water

flesh and water of 1 young coconut
1 tablespoon raw cacao powder
1 tablespoon maca powder
1 cup berries, any variety
greens

1 banana

2 pears

2 tablespoons macadamia nut butter

1½ cups water

greens

¼ cup diced beets

¼ cup hemp seeds

¼ cup goji berries, soaked overnight (optional)

1½ cups water

greens

---

1 Lebanese cucumber

I cup strawberries

4 dried figs soaked in 1 cup water (reserve and add the water)

1 to 2 tablespoons chia seeds

greens

---

2 cups cubed pineapple with core

I lime, peeled

½ avocado

1½ cups water

watercress

---

2 bananas

inner leaf gel of 4 inches aloe vera

1 teaspoon vanilla extract

1½ cups pumpkinseed milk

1 tablespoon melted coconut oil

greens

---

1 mango

1 orange, peeled

1½ cups juiced burdock root and celery

greens

⅛ cup oat groats, soaked

1 cup red berries (any variety)

1 pear

1½ cups water or nut milk

greens

sweetener, as needed

---

1 cup durian flesh

1 banana

½ to 1 teaspoon ground cinnamon

1 to 2 teaspoons raw cacao powder (optional)

1 teaspoon vanilla extract

1½ cups water

greens

I cup frozen unhulled strawberries

1 cup raspberries

1½ cups water

4 tablespoons hemp seeds

zest of ½ lemon

borage flowers and leaves or other mild, pale greens (so the smoothie stays nice and pink!)

---

1 cup blueberries

½ avocado

1 banana

1 to 2 tablespoons raw cacao powder

2 teaspoons micro-algae

greens

Mood

Our mood and mental health are reliant upon many factors that can be influenced by excellent nutrition. For our brain to work well so we feel good and smart, we need our neurotransmitters to do their job quickly and efficiently. Neurotransmitters are the messengers between the ends of two nerves, the meeting place being a synapse. Nerves need to communicate with each other extremely quickly, and if our neurotransmitters aren't working, we don't function properly.

Our brain is 60 percent fat, so it needs to be fed with good-quality fats such as omega-3 and -6 fatty acids and saturated fats from coconut. We need vitamin B5 and choline to help make the very important neurotransmitter acetylcholine. We need vitamin B6 and the amino acid tryptophan to help make serotonin. We need the amino acid tyrosine to help make adrenaline and dopamine. Further, all of the B vitamins, vitamin C, folic acid, zinc, and magnesium are essential for our brain.

Good blood sugar balance is also essential for our mood, assisted by (in addition to a low-glycemic, whole-food diet), vitamin C, folic acid, zinc, magnesium, and chromium. So our green smoothie–friendly mood and brain foods can include:

• Pumpkin, sunflower, sesame, and chia seeds for zinc

- Romaine lettuce, tomatoes, apples, bananas, nettles, and grape juice for chromium
- Pumpkinseeds, chia seeds, raw cacao, almonds, cashews, bananas, beet greens, and spinach for magnesium
- Avocado, banana, sunflower seeds, walnuts, and spinach for vitamin B6
- Spinach and oranges for folic acid
- Lecithin and sunflower seeds for choline
- Cinnamon and cilantro for assistance with insulin regulation
- Chia and micro-algae for complete protein and omega-3 sources (especially marine phytoplankton)
- Flax, walnuts, hemp seed, and purslane for extra omega-3 and -6 essential fats
- Sesame, spirulina, and spinach for tryptophan, and spirulina for tyrosine
- Lots of fresh raw fruits and tender herbs for vitamin C, and dried fruits like apricots, figs, and dates for extra B vitamins. Vitamin C not only aids absorption of iron, but chromium, too.

For a bit of bliss, don't forget PEA (phenylethylamine), the "love chemical" present in AFA blue-green algae, and cherries, which contain the tryptamine "melatonin," a relaxation and sleep aid. Cacao activates tryptamines, so combined, your green smoothie will have a chocolate-cherry theme that should result in a very "chilled out" effect. Perhaps this is a better green smoothie for evening?

Mood-Enhancing Green Smoothies

Water or coconut water can be substituted for nut and seed milks:

1 banana

I pear

1 apple

2 tablespoons chia seeds

1 teaspoon ground cinnamon

1 teaspoon vanilla extract

1½ cups sunflower seed milk

greens

....

1 banana

1 cup berries, any variety

2 tablespoons high omega-3 oil

1½ cups water

mint

....

3 to 4 oranges, peeled

½ avocado

1½ cups sesame milk

cilantro

....

1 lemon, quartered

zest of 1 lemon

1 orange, peeled

1 banana

1½ cups orange juice

parsley

....

1 cup apricots

1 banana

1 tablespoon soy lecithin or organic sunflower oil

1½ cups almond milk

greens

....

1 cup ripe tomatoes

½ avocado

1½ cups fennel juice and/or celery juice

basil and mint

2 cups red grapes

¼ cup hemp seeds

1 teaspoon ground cinnamon

1½ cups water

greens

1 cup dried figs soaked overnight (discard water)

1 inch fresh ginger

1 small banana

1½ cups walnut milk

greens

Fall in love with this smoothie as it contains high levels of PEA, the "love chemical," present in the AFA algae and cacao:

2 bananas

2 Medjool dates

2 to 3 tablespoons hemp seeds

2 tablespoons raw cacao powder

2 teaspoons AFA algae

1½ cups water

greens

In this green smoothie, the magnesium in the chia, cashews, and cacao, and the cacao-activated melatonin in cherries are bound to totally chill you out.

1½ cup pitted cherries

2 tablespoons raw cacao powder

2 tablespoons chia seeds

2 cups cashew milk

greens

Be chilled and be in love with this supercharged mood smoothie!

1 cup pitted cherries

1 banana

2 tablespoons raw cacao powder

2 teaspoons AFA algae

1 cup cashew milk

½ cup ice cubes

2 tablespoons hemp seeds

greens

Featured Recipe

Sandy Forster (www.wildlywealthywomen.com) is an award-winning entrepreneur, international prosperity mentor, and worldwide adventurer. She is the author of the bestseller *How to Be Wildly Wealthy FAST*. Sandy walks the talk when it comes to nurturing her health, and this mood-boosting smoothie must be the secret to her success!

1 frozen banana, sliced

½ cup shredded coconut

1 orange, peeled

handful of goji berries

2 tablespoons chia seeds

30 fresh spearmint leaves

2 kale leaves

2 cups parsley

dash of ground cinnamon

stevia, as needed

1½ cups spring water

Says Sandy, "I am so hooked on my latest green smoothie—supersonically good for me and straight out of my own veggie patch! So yummy!"

Fertility and Maternal Health

Pre-Conception and Pregnancy

The health of a child starts before and during pregnancy. Nutrients like vitamins B6 and B12, folic acid, choline, zinc, magnesium, iron, probiotics, and essential fats are important for the mother-to-be for her own health and that of the growing baby. From pre-conception care though breastfeeding, green smoothies are a fabulous way of delivering nutrition.

Zinc, magnesium, and iron can be found in pumpkinseeds, sesame seeds, and chia seeds. Iron is also found in apricots, peaches, figs, avocados, and leafy greens like spinach, chard, and romaine lettuce. Magnesium is also found in almonds, Brazil nuts, cashews, bananas, figs, beet greens, and spinach. Cacao is super rich in magnesium, but the stimulating properties of raw cacao should be kept to a minimum for pregnant women, particularly in the first trimester. Folic acid is found in leafy greens and oranges, and vitamin B6 is found in avocado, bananas, sunflower seeds, spinach, and walnuts. Soy lecithin and sunflower oil contain choline. Enzyme-rich and tonifying alfalfa is safe to use during pregnancy and is great for breastfeeding women.

Beneficial fats include omega-3 and -6 fatty acids, such as alpha-linolenic acid (ALA) found in chia seeds, hemp seeds, walnuts, and purslane. Gamma-linolenic acid (GLA) is an anti-inflammatory omega-6 oil found in breast milk and also in spirulina, hemp, borage, and evening primrose. ALA is also in AFA algae and chlorella, and eicosapentaenoic acid (EPA) and docosahexaenoic acid are in marine phytoplankton. Coconut oil aids the absorption of essential fatty acids and assists the conversion of ALA to EPA and DHA in the body. Coconut oil is also rich in lauric acid, the predominant fatty acid in breast milk.

Ginger and herbs such as parsley, mint, cilantro, and basil have essential oils that are soothing to the stomach and may be beneficial in green smoothies if a pregnant woman is prone to nausea. Furthermore, green smoothies made with nut milk bases and with fewer ingredients taste less acidic and are more likely to be well received by the stomach.

Pregnant women with blood sugar issues such as gestational diabetes may benefit from the regular use of cilantro and cinnamon in their green smoothies.

Gabriela Rosa is a leading clinician, author, and internationally recognized naturopath and fertility specialist. Rosa is a huge fan of eating nutrient-dense foods, including green smoothies. This is what she has to say about fertility:

> A healthy body is a fertile body, but optimum
> fertility means much more than just being able to
> achieve conception and deliver a healthy baby at term.
> By eight weeks gestation, a baby's health blueprint is

already created, as are his or her tiny organs and little fingerprints! At this stage his or her health vulnerabilities and strengths are set by the "map" already existent in this magnificent design—your child's future health predispositions and potentials are now in place regardless of what else happens from this point onwards, and most parents-to-be are unaware of this crucial fact. Once a pregnancy is established, your child's health potential becomes the lowest common denominator of you and your partner's health at that point and its full potential has been reached—the opportunity for making significant improvements to your fertility and your child's health in the future exists in the 120 days of pre-conception preparation before a pregnancy is even in sight. The time to optimize your child's future, giving him or her the best possible start in life is NOT during your pregnancy—it is during your pre-conception preparation, involving both prospective parents.

Of course you can make a difference to your child's health during gestation by the many things you do and the ways in which you conduct yourself. So eating and deriving sustenance and real nutrition from your daily food choices is essential and paramount for optimum results—if you are planning for a healthy baby, remember to act pregnant by eating like you're pregnant, for at least 120 days prior to a conception attempt, to get pregnant later. This is the approximate amount of time it takes for the egg to mature and the sperm that will be the originating cells of your child's future to form. Focus your love and attention to this task and you will be able to rest assured you have done your very best for creating a truly healthy baby.

Rosa's top fertility foods are:
* coconut water and flesh—full of nutrients, electrolytes, and fats that are essential building blocks for hormones and cells
* cilantro, parsley, and mint—all high in nutrients and chlorophyll, excellent for detoxifying
* garlic—great for immunity and as an anti-clotting cardiovascular health booster
* artichoke—wonderful liver tonic and detoxifier
* bitter melon—fantastic blood sugar regulator
* avocado—fabulous essential fatty acids
* berries—full of antioxidant anthocyanins

Leafy greens are also considered excellent for fertility due to their high level of nutrition and alkalinity. However, Rosa recommends avoiding potentially goitrogenic greens like kale and cabbages. Goitrogens may interfere with the thyroid's ability to take up iodine. Iodine is necessary for a healthy thryroid and a healthy thyroid is necessary for fertility.

Recipes for Before and During Pregnancy

Where "greens" are listed, aim to include spinach, chard, beet greens, romaine lettuce, alfalfa sprouts, and borage (include the flowers, stems, and leaves).

Water or coconut water can be substituted for nut milks. The daily addition of micro-algae such as marine phytoplankton (for DHA) and spirulina (for GLA) is highly recommended:

1½ cups sunflower seed or pumpkinseed milk

2 to 3 bananas

mint and borage

1 mango

1 inch fresh ginger

1½ cups coconut water

cilantro and spinach

2 to 3 bananas

1 tablespoon soy lecithin or organic sunflower oil

1½ cups water

greens

2 oranges, peeled

1 to 2 tablespoons hemp seeds

1½ cups cashew milk

greens

1 banana

1 small avocado

zest of ½ lemon

1½ cups water

parsley and spinach

1½ cups apricots

½ teaspoon ground cinnamon

1 teaspoon vanilla extract

1½ cups almond milk

greens

2 bananas

1 teaspoon ground cinnamon or Instant Chai Spice Mix (page 230)

1 tablespoon chia seeds

1½ cups sesame milk

greens

2 large peaches

1 to 2 tablespoons chia seeds

1 inch fresh ginger

1½ cups almond milk

greens

4 fresh figs

½ small avocado

1½ cups walnut or pecan milk

cilantro and spinach

2 bananas

I peach or 2 apricots

1 inch fresh ginger

1½ cups Brazil nut milk

greens

Fertility-Boosting Recipes

1 cup mixed berries

flesh and water of 1 Thai coconut

mint

3 peaches

½ cup raspberries

1½ cups almond milk

spinach

2 bananas

2 cups unhulled strawberries

1 cup coconut water

cilantro

½ cup prepared raw baby artichoke leaves*

1 small garlic clove

1 cup tomatoes

flesh of 1 medium lemon

3 tablespoons olive oil

parsley

salt and pepper, as needed

* *To prepare the artichoke leaves, cut off the artichoke's stem and break off the outer tough leaves. Slice 1 inch off the tips of the leaves and remove the fuzzy core. Cut into quarters, and if not using immediately, rub lemon juice over the cut sides.*

½ prepared bitter melon*

zest and flesh of 1 lemon

½ avocado

2 cups apple juice

spinach

* *To prepare the bitter melon, scrape and cut it in half lengthwise. Remove the seeds and thinly slice. Salt the flesh and set aside for 10 to 15 minutes to reduce the bitterness of the melon. Wash with plenty of water. Drain and squeeze out any excess water.*

Babies and Children

Babies

Green smoothies can be introduced to children at six months old, or when they start to eat solids. Given that the contents are blended, digestion of green smoothies is easier than food that needs to be chewed. Fruits for smoothies are the same as those that are normally introduced to a baby first, like banana, mango, papaya, and peaches. Here they're blended with a small amount of mild greens. Avoid stronger and bitter greens until the child is much older, but just like in smoothies for adults, the greens should be rotated regularly. It's also very important for a child's development to eat healthy fats, so the addition of avocado or coconut works very well. Some foods should ideally be introduced after a child is a year old, or even two years if the child has a sensitive digestive system. These foods include potentially allergenic foods like oranges, nuts, and seeds, and high-pectin fruits that are harder for developing digestive systems to eat raw, such as sour apples and berries, citrus peel and most unripe fruits, which are better left uneaten or cooked.

To make 1 cup (250 mL) of green smoothie for a baby, combine:

½ cup water, coconut water, or a combination

½ cup 1 to 2 chopped fruits like banana, papaya, mango, and peaches, or ½ cup chopped 1 fruit and some avocado or young coconut flesh

¼ cup loosely packed greens like spinach, kale, bok choy, butter lettuce, radish tops, or romaine

This amount may be fed over more than one meal in a day.

Children over 2 Years Old

Children raised on green smoothies from a young age tend to want and ask for green smoothies as they get older. Children who are introduced to green smoothies at an older age may be fussy with the taste and the color.

The best thing is not to make a big deal about what you are feeding them. Try using cups that are not clear or cups with lids and straws. Make the smoothies purple with blueberries, or make a brown smoothie and say its chocolate, or make it pink using strawberries and raspberries with a light-colored green like bok choy. Get your kids involved in making their smoothies. Give the smoothies funny names and make a game of it, such as drawing the names of the smoothies on a big piece of paper that is displayed in the kitchen. Avoid stronger and bitter greens until your child is much older.

To make 2 cups (500 mL) of green smoothie for your child, combine:

1 cup water, coconut water, nut milk, or a combination

1 cup 1 to 2 chopped fruits, like banana, papaya, mango, peaches, apricots, avocado, oranges, mandarin oranges, berries, ripe pears, sweet apples, and pineapple

½ cup loosely packed greens, like spinach, kale, bok choy, butter lettuce, radish tops, or romaine

Probiotics

Probiotics are essential for a healthy immune system with pregnant women, and mothers who use them frequently report better energy and less illness for themselves and their children. Probiotics are ideal to use during pre-conception, pregnancy, and breastfeeding, and they can can be given to children and even bottle-fed babies.

Banana-less Green Smoothies

The humble banana is a staple for many green smoothie drinkers; some people claim to eat as many as 30 bananas a day! Others prefer not to eat fruit that is commercially hybridized, or avoid bananas because they're high glycemic. Some people just don't like bananas.

I am a definite fan of bananas. They provide a creamy texture and richness to a smoothie that is hard to re-create, especially using frozen bananas, which add an ice-cream quality to a smoothie. However, I have been challenged by others to create recipes without bananas, and I had no choice in 2011 in Australia, as tropical cyclone Yasi tore through Queensland and decimated most of our banana industry. Paying twenty dollars for six bananas is not my idea of fun, so making smoothies without them over an Australian winter was an interesting and successful challenge.

Without a fruit or ingredient that creates thickness, the smoothie will be more like a thick juice and will likely not be filling enough. This is important if your smoothie is your meal, such as breakfast. Instead, to thicken a banana-less smoothie, use fruits rich in soluble fiber, such as:

- apples (with skin)
- berries (fresh or frozen)
- chia seeds
- citrus (whole, peeled)
- kiwifruit
- mangoes
- pears (with skin)
- plums
- strawberries

Frozen berries are available all year round, and blueberries are great because they don't have the tiny seeds that can get stuck in your teeth. Surprisingly, blueberries can thicken up your smoothie not unlike chia seeds do. Chia seeds are another great way to add bulk to your green smoothie if it is a bit too thin. Either pre-soak the seeds in water to form a gel or add dry seeds to the smoothie; they will break down either way. Aim for 1 to 2 tablespoons per smoothie.

To add creaminess, a source of fat works well, such as avocado, hemp seeds, walnut oil, or coconut flesh. For any smoothie that is not sweet enough, you can always add a sweetener of your choice.

Banana-less Spring Recipes

1½ cups cantaloupe

I cup unhulled strawberries

1 cup water

greens

1 cup whole kumquats

1 apple

1 Lebanese cucumber

1 teaspoon vanilla extract

1 cup water

parsley

2 oranges, peeled

I lime, peeled

½ avocado

1½ cups orange juice

watercress

1 cup star fruit

½ cup young coconut flesh

1½ cups coconut water

cilantro

1 cup pink grapefruit, peeled

2 mandarin oranges, peeled

zest and flesh of I lemon

½ avocado

greens

sweetener, as needed

Banana-less Summer Recipes

2 cups apricots

½ teaspoon ground cinnamon

¼ teaspoon ground cardamom

1 teaspoon vanilla extract

1½ cups almond milk

greens

1½ cups berries

flesh and water of 1 young coconut

small handful of basil leaves

spinach

1½ cups grapes (any variety)

2 cups melon (any variety)

greens

1 mango

2 oranges, peeled

Banana-less Autumn Recipes

4 fresh figs

1 cup raspberries

1½ cups water or nut milk

basil

spinach

1½ cups honeydew melon

1 cup green grapes

1 cup water

mint or other greens

3 pears

1 teaspoon ground cinnamon

⅛ teaspoon ground clove

½ teaspoon ground cardamom

1 inch fresh ginger

1 teaspoon vanilla

1½ cups almond milk

greens

2 to 3 nectarines

flesh of 2 lemons

zest of 1 lemon

1 inch fresh ginger

1½ cups water

greens

sweetener, as needed

---

3 oranges, peeled

juice of 1 large or 2 small pomegranates*

1 cup water or nut milk

parsley

* To juice pomegranates, peel and blend whole, then strain
  through a nut milk bag or cheesecloth.

Banana-less Winter Recipes

1 cup tamarillo flesh

¼ cup raisins, soaked overnight

1 teaspoon vanilla extract

1½ cups almond milk

greens

---

flesh and water of 1 young coconut

1 cup pineapple with core

1 inch fresh ginger

greens

½ cup young coconut flesh

juice of 1 large or 2 small pomegranates*

2 cups walnut milk or 2 cups water with 2 tablespoons walnut oil

greens

* To juice pomegranates, peel and blend whole, then strain
  through a nut milk bag or cheesecloth.

Featured Recipe

Dr. Ritamarie Loscalzo (www.greensmoothiecleanse.com) is a leading authority on nutrition and health. She's an author, speaker, and health practitioner with over two decades of experience empowering health through education, inspiration, and loving care. This delicious green smoothie is her staple recipe:

1 cup mango, fresh or frozen

1 cup pineapple, fresh or frozen

1 cup papaya, fresh or frozen

water and flesh of 1 fresh young coconut

1 inch fresh ginger

juice of 1 lemon or 2 limes

as many greens as possible

---

2 pears

1 apple

½ teaspoon grated or ground nutmeg

1½ cups almond milk

kale or cabbage

4 oranges and/or tangelos, peeled

1 cup fennel juice

1 to 2 tablespoons chia seeds

fennel tops

1 cup water

greens

passion fruit flesh, to top each serving

1½ cups peeled, seeded lychees

1½ cups almond milk

mint

Fructose-Friendly Smoothies

A diagnosis of fructose malabsorption can be frustrating when everyday foods such as honey, onions, garlic, apples, and pears cannot be eaten anymore. This condition is due to the body's inability to absorb fructose through the small intestine, where it would usually be taken to the liver for metabolism. Instead, an abnormal amount of fructose remains in the intestines where it ferments, causing abdominal discomfort or pain, gas, bloating, diarrhea, or constipation. It can present like and co-exist with irritable bowel syndrome.

The diet for this condition includes eliminating foods containing fructans (long chains of fructose molecules) and foods that have a high ratio of fructose to glucose.

Usual green smoothie–friendly ingredients that are *not* allowed are: apples, pears, watermelon, guava, honeydew melon, mango, nashi fruit (Asian pear), papaya, quince, star fruit, cherry, grape, persimmon, lychee, dried fruits, coconut, honey, and agave nectar. Any fruit juice concentrates, fruit pastes, jams, and canned fruits and fruit juices are also not allowed.

Green smoothie ingredients that are allowed are:

- Stone fruit: apricot, nectarine, peach, plum
- Berry fruit: blueberry, blackberry, boysenberry, cranberry, raspberry, strawberry
- Citrus fruit: kumquat, grapefruit, lemon, lime, mandarin orange, orange, tangelo
- Other fruits: ripe banana, jackfruit, kiwifruit, passion fruit, pineapple, tamarillo

There seems to be variable consensus about nuts, leafy greens, and sweeteners such as stevia, raw sugar, and sugar alcohols like xylitol. To stay as simple as possible, in the following recipes I have not used any extra sweeteners, nuts or nut milks, and specific greens are not indicated. If you have fructose malabsorption, you likely know what you can and cannot have, depending on sensitivity.

Fructose-Friendly Recipes

2 bananas
1 cup berries
1½ cups water
greens

1 banana
½ medium pineapple with core
1½ cups water
greens

2 cups sweet citrus, peeled
I cup blueberries
2 tablespoons chia seeds
1 cup water
greens

1 cup apricots or peaches
I banana
½ teaspoon ground cardamom
½ teaspoon ground cinnamon
1 teaspoon vanilla extract
1½ cups water
greens

3 bananas
½ teaspoon grated or ground nutmeg
I teaspoon vanilla extract
1½ cups water
greens

1 cup tamarillo flesh and seeds
flesh and zest of ½ lime
1 avocado
1½ cups water
greens

2 cups of sweet citrus, peeled
½ avocado
I pink grapefruit, peeled
1 peach
1½ cups water
greens

2 bananas
zest of 1 lemon
1 cup raspberries
1½ cups water
greens

1 Lebanese cucumber

1 cup unhulled strawberries

1 kiwifruit (include the skin for extra fiber)

1 cup water

greens

2 kiwifruit

I orange, peeled

1 inch fresh ginger

1 avocado

1½ cups water

greens

flesh of 1 to 2 passion fruits, stirred through the finished smoothies

½ medium pineapple with core

1 lime, peeled

2 tablespoons chia seeds

Fussy About Fruit

I have a friend whose digestive system is super sensitive to fiber yet tormented by wanting to eat fruit and greens for nutritional reasons. This friend is also severely hypoglycemic, so she needs higher protein in a smoothie to sustain her. After some trial and error, we found these smoothies that work for both her conditions, and most importantly, they allow her to eat blended greens and fruit without distress. She has found that blended greens are far easier for her to digest than if she chews them; a poorly blended smoothie is no good either. The thicker the smoothie, the better: if it's too thin, it will digest too quickly and contribute to diarrhea.

If you wish to follow a low-fructose or low-sugar diet, then these green smoothies are appropriate as long as you are not vegan or dairy intolerant. These recipes do have an animal product base rather than a plant or water base, and use only a small amount of fruit with a good fructose to glucose ratio.

Combine one of the following fruit options:

½ large banana, ½ small mango, ⅔ cup any berries, 1 large peach, 2 apricots, or 1 large nectarine

and

1 cup good-quality probiotic dairy yogurt, sheep or goat yogurt, or dairy kefir

and

1 to 2 scoops whey protein powder, or Sunwarrior Raw Vegan Protein Powder or, 1 to 2 raw organic, free-range eggs

and

¾ to 1 cup of greens

¼ teaspoon whole-leaf stevia

1 tsp of cinnamon

Superfoods

Superfoods are super-nutritious—they contain not just one nutrient or a few nutrients, but many. I aim to use what I call super whole foods. My top 10 are not all smoothie friendly, although most are. They include quinoa, chia seeds, sea vegetables, coconut, lemon, beets, lentils, leafy greens, avocado, and berries. These whole foods are bursting with nutrition and are easily added to my diet generally to ensure that I consume plenty of vitamins, minerals, antioxidants, essentials fats, and all essential amino acids.

I am also a fan of food-based superfood formulas and powders such as maca powder, raw cacao powder, Gubinge (Kakadu plum, very high in vitamin C), micro-algae, In-Liven Fermented Probiotic Superfood, Berry Radical Antioxidant Superfood, and medicinal mushrooms.

Other green smoothie–friendly superfoods include lucuma powder, mesquite powder, noni, goji berries, acai and maqui berries, mangosteen, bee pollen, and hemp seeds.

Any extra superfoods can be added to a green smoothie, however, sometimes they affect the taste. For example, raw cacao, mesquite powder, maca, and noni are strong in flavor, algae and berry powders have minimal to moderate taste, while probiotics and high–vitamin C powders have no taste. The challenge with the stronger-flavored superfoods is using small amounts, finding flavor combinations that mask or complement, or just putting up with a smoothie that may well be borderline unpleasant.

Most people who are regular smoothie drinkers, especially for breakfast, will use their smoothie as their superfood and supplement delivery device. At a minimum I always put In-Liven Probiotic in my green smoothie, and at times I may add as many as four or five other items, including bee pollen, antioxidant powders, colloidal minerals like silica or magnesium, vitamin C powders, and micro-algae. What I put in changes over time depending on what I feel I need, what time I have, what I want my smoothie to taste like, and what I have available. There are no rules!

Superfood-Packed Recipes

¼ cup goji berries, soaked

1 cup fresh or frozen berries

1 tablespoon raw cacao powder

flesh and water of 1 young coconut

1 tablespoon melted coconut oil (add last)

greens

2 bananas

½ avocado

2 tablespoons raw cacao powder

2 teaspoons AFA algae

1½ cups water

greens

¼ cup cubed beet

1 cup pitted cherries

zest of ½ lemon

½ avocado

1½ cups nut or seed milk

greens

2 bananas

flesh of 1 young coconut

1 tablespoon raw honey

1 tablespoon bee pollen

1½ cups water

greens

1 cup berries

1 orange, peeled

4 tablespoons hemp seeds

1½ cups water

greens

1 banana

2 tablespoons chia seeds

1 teaspoon ground cinnamon

2 teaspoons vanilla extract

1 tablespoon maca powder

3 cups almond milk

mild greens

¼ cup diced beets

2 pears

1 tablespoon raw cacao powder

4 tablespoon hemp seeds

1½ cups water or nut/seed milk

greens

1 banana

1 cup pineapple with core

2 teaspoons of micro-algae

1½ cups water

cilantro

1 tablespoon soy lecithin

2 to 3 bananas

1 teaspoon ground cinnamon

2 teaspoons mesquite powder

1½ cups sunflower seed milk

greens

flesh and water of 1 young coconut

1 lemon, quartered

1 tablespoon raw honey

1 tablespoon lucuma powder

greens

2 cups pitted cherries

1 tablespoon maqui or acai berry powder

1½ cups seed milk

greens

Featured Recipe

David "Avocado" Wolfe (www.davidwolfe.com), to most who have heard of him, is a raw food and superfood expert. However, what you may not know is that David has a master's degree in nutrition and a background in science and mechanical engineering. He is considered one of the world's top authorities on natural health, beauty, nutrition, herbalism, chocolate, and organic superfoods. David is a highly sought after health and personal-success speaker, having given over 2000 live lectures since the late 1990s! I personally met David as part of his Australian tour in 2010 and 2011, and he was simply inspiring to be around and to listen to.

David has kindly provided his Superfood Berry Green Smoothie:

½ cup of blueberries

½ cup of raspberries

handful of goji berries

flesh and water of 1 young coconut

1 tablespoon raw cacao powder

1 tablespoon maca powder

1 tablespoon hemp seeds

1 tablespoon reishi mushroom powder (mycelium)

inner leaf gel of a 4-inch square piece of aloe vera inner leaf gel (or equivalent size)

spirulina and/or E3Live AFA blue-green algae and/or marine phytoplankton (dose according to bottle)*

leafy greens of choice

½ to 1 cup spring water

raw wild honey, to sweeten

Blend all the ingredients except the spring water and honey. Add the spring water as needed until the desired consistency is reached. Add the honey a little at a time until the balance of sweetness is right.

*David advises using spirulina during the warmer months of the year (as spirulina is cooling), and blue-green algae and/or marine phytoplankton during the cooler months (as they are warming).

Blended Green Juices

I often hear that people want the benefits of green smoothies, namely the fiber, but they don't want to drink a full smoothie, which is very filling. I completely agree, as I struggle to drink a quart of green smoothie daily. I consume half a quart of green smoothie for breakfast, but I really like to *eat* lunch and dinner. However, I do want the super-nutrition a full quart can provide.

The solution that works for me is blending plain greens into juice, blending greens with very juicy fruits like watermelon, or blending a small amount of fruit with water and greens. I will tend to drink these juices prior to lunch and dinner, and the drinks often contain lemon as a digestive aid for my meal.

You can use a traditional juicer to make juice and then use a blender to blend fresh greens through it. Any liquid base can be used in this instance, be it actual juice, water, coconut water, or nut milk. Moreover, blended green juices are a great way of using vegetables that don't work as well in a smoothie, such as fennel, celery, carrots, and beets.

If you want to use ice in your green juice, a heavy-duty blender such as a Thermomix, Blendtec, or Vitamix is best. Ice will help keep the temperature of the blended liquid down in the Vitamix or Blendtec, although it is not necessary in a Thermomix.

Blended Juice Recipes

If using ice, reduce the amount of liquid proportionally:

3½ cups pineapple and cucumber juice

mint

spinach

---

3 cups watermelon

½ cup water

greens

I lemon, quartered

zest of 1 lemon

3½ cups apple juice

parsley

½ cup blueberries

3½ cups orange or tangelo juice

greens

3½ cups fennel and apple juice

fennel tops

spinach

3½ cups celery, carrot, and beet juice

greens

---

2 teaspoons Instant Chai Spice Mix (page 230)

2 cups carrot juice

1½ cups nut milk

borage leaves

3½ cups sweetened vanilla nut milk

bok choy or radish tops

greens

----

1 inch fresh ginger

3½ cups cucumber juice

greens

3½ cups coconut water

greens

This final green smoothie recipe is about 55 percent coconut water and 45 percent greens. Blood is made up plasma and blood cells. Plasma comprises 55 percent of blood fluid and is mostly water (90 percent by volume), and contains dissolved proteins, glucose, mineral ions, hormones, carbon dioxide, platelets, and red and white blood cells. Red blood cells are the most abundant and they contain hemoglobin, an iron-containing protein. The plant version of hemoglobin is chlorophyll, a green pigment based around a magnesium ion as opposed to iron (heme). Both hemoglobin and chlorophyll exist to obtain energy. Coconut water is the natural liquid closest in structure to blood plasma and has been used in times of war instead of plasma when supplies were low. This is all a very scientific way of saying that by combining 55 percent coconut water and 45 percent greens, and you'll have a BLOODy great green smoothie!

Simple and Stunning

Green smoothies can get very complicated. They can have so many ingredients that the end result is a mishmash of undistinguishable flavor. If you are like me and you want your green smoothies to:

1. Taste great
2. Have a minimal number of ingredients
3. Taste like the ingredients you put in them

Then these smoothies are for you.

Simple Smoothie Recipes

Unless otherwise specified, use about 1½ to 2 cups fruit to coconut flesh, 1½ cups water or nut milk, and any variety of greens in the desired quantity.

banana

coconut water

greens

strawberries

young coconut flesh

water

greens

sweetener, as needed

---

peaches

raspberries

water

greens

3½ cups watermelon

mint

greens

(no water or nut milk)

---

pineapple

banana

water

mint

---

banana

1 to 2 teaspoons Instant Chai Spice Mix (page 230)

nut milk

greens

---

oranges

mango

water

greens

---

red papaya

banana

water

greens

banana

1 to 2 tablespoons raw cacao powder

water

mint

---

whole lemons

honey

water

greens

---

cantaloupe

water

greens

---

mandarins

4 tablespoons hemp seeds

water

greens

---

banana

blueberries

water

greens

---

3 cups honeydew melon

½ cup ice cubes

mint

greens

And this, I believe, is the sexiest simple green smoothie ever…

2 frozen bananas, sliced

1 mango

water from 1 young Thai coconut

1 teaspoon vanilla extract

Swiss chard or spinach

Savory

For anyone wishing to get the benefits of blending greens without using sweet fruit, then savory green smoothies are the way to go. This may be due to the need or desire to reduce sugar consumption for weight or candida management. These smoothies may feel most natural to eat for lunch or dinner.

These green smoothies could also be called raw soups, and can be made thicker so they can be eaten with a spoon. To make them thicker, use less water, more greens, or add chia seeds and let it sit for up to an hour to thicken.

Some of these recipes use ice to help incorporate the more fibrous veggies into these savory green smoothies. If you prefer a slightly warmed savory smoothie, blend longer than usual, about 3 minutes, so the friction of the blender starts to warm it up. If you have a Thermomix, it won't warm with friction, so set it to the 37°C button (98°F) for a few minutes to warm it up and still retain the enzymes.

Savory Recipes

Try these savory green smoothies or soups at any time of the day:

1 cup ripe tomatoes

1 avocado

1½ cups fennel and/or celery juice

4 sprigs basil

handful of spinach

---

2 sun-dried tomatoes, soaked

2 cups tomatoes

1 small lemon, peeled

½ cup ice cubes

½ cup water

3 ribs celery, top half (with leaves) only

splash of Bragg's Liquid Aminos or tamari

pinch cayenne pepper

cracked black pepper

---

1 cup yellow cherry tomatoes

1 yellow bell pepper

½ avocado

¼ teaspoon ground turmeric

pinch of cayenne pepper

squeeze of lemon juice

1½ cups water

6 pieces green stem bok choy or 3 to 4 leaves Napa cabbage/
wombok

½ cup sugar snap peas

1 avocado

juice of ½ lemon

½ cup ice cubes

1 cup water

1 to 2 handfuls pea greens

pinch salt

2 to 3 sprigs of mint

¼ cup diced beets

1 Granny Smith apple

⅛ medium red onion

juice of ½ lemon

1½ cups water

½ cup ice cubes

2 tablespoons tahini

1 bunch of cilantro

---

1 cup tomatoes

1 red bell pepper

½ clove garlic

1½ cups water

2 tablespoons olive oil

a sprig of rosemary

a sprig of oregano

a good handful of parsley

salt and pepper, as needed

½ teaspoon ground fennel seeds

1 small fennel bulb with tops

1 Lebanese cucumber

zest of ½ orange or lemon

juice 1 orange

3 tablespoons olive oil

1 cup water

½ cup ice

1 sprig tarragon

1 to 2 handfuls spinach or Swiss chard

¼ teaspoon salt

pinch of cracked black pepper

Use 1½ cups of water and stevia as needed for a totally fruit-free smoothie

1 cup diced celery root

1 Granny Smith apple

1½ cups almond milk

½ cup ice cubes

1 bunch parsley

pinch of salt and pepper

1 avocado

1 Lebanese cucumber

zest of 1 lime

2 limes, peeled

1½ cups water

2 handfuls watercress or 4 to 5 kale leaves

stevia, as needed if tart or bitter

Featured Recipe

Leisa Wheeler, the founder of Embracing Health (www.embracinghealth
.com.au), is a naturopath who specializes in hormonal fatigue disorders.
She runs six-day detox, healing, and raw food retreats in Bali and
Australia, and uses green smoothies as part of her program. This is
one of her favorite savory green smoothies:

½ cup arugula

½ cup watercress

1 cup kale

1 cucumber

1 carrot

1 beet

2 ribs celery

½ lemon

pinch of cayenne pepper

pinch of Celtic sea salt

splash of tamari

2 cups water

3 tablespoons chia seeds

1 cup carrot juice

1 cup almond milk

1 cup ice

1 bunch cilantro

pinch of salt

Just Desserts

Who says green smoothies can't be a decadent experience reminiscent of a restaurant dessert or sweet café snack? Despite our dairy-free and gluten-free diet, my English husband still pines over the possibility of eating banoffee pie (an English cream pie made with toffee and bananas) and cheesecake. The following recipes are dedicated to my husband and other dessert fans who just can't imagine a life without sweets.

All of these recipes are rich and creamy. For the smoothie to still taste like dessert, mild greens like spinach or Swiss chard are usually called for, and not in a huge quantity. If you wish the color not to come out green, for example, a pink color for "Strawberry Cheesecake," then a mild and pale green is required. Pale mild greens include green baby bok choy, radish tops, borage leaves and flowers, butter lettuce, collards, and napa cabbage. I know this a bit of a gimmick, but it's a lot of fun! All recipes make 2 medium to large glasses or four small glasses.

Banoffee Pie

3 to 4 frozen bananas

2 Medjool dates, soaked overnight, or 2 tablespoons maple syrup

4 teaspoons mesquite powder

1½ cups almond milk

pale, mild greens

Blend and serve with a sprinkle of mesquite powder.

Tiramisu

1½ cups cooled strong teeccino brew (or other caffeine-free coffee substitute)

2 frozen, sliced pears

1 cup Raw Vanilla Ice Cream (page 229)

1 tablespoon raw cacao powder

mild greens

Blend and top with shaved chocolate.

Strawberry Cheesecake

½ cup raw macadamias

1 cup frozen, halved, unhulled strawberries

1 cup of strawberries, dehydrated

1½ cups young Thai coconut water

zest of half a lemon

pale, mild greens

Blend and garnish with a big, fresh strawberry on the glass.

Black Forest Cake

1½ cups frozen blueberries or pitted cherries

1 cup Raw Vanilla Ice Cream (page 229)

2 tablespoons raw cacao powder

4 soaked, Medjool dates or 4 tablespoons agave, honey, or maple syrup

1 cup hazelnut milk

2 teaspoons vanilla extract

pinch of salt

greens

Blend and drizzle the top with raw chocolate ganache.

For Raw Chocolate Ganache:

¼ cup raw cacao powder

¼ cup honey, agave, or maple syrup

¼ cup melted coconut oil

good of pinch of salt

Stir together the cacao and sweetener, then stir in the oil. Larger or smaller quantities can be made keeping the ratios the same. Ganache will keep without needing refrigeration; it needs to be over 76°F (24°C) to be liquid and will be hard below 65°F (18°C).

You can also top the smoothie with Loving Earth's Raw Organic Coconut Chocolate Butter.

Lemon Tart

2 frozen bananas

½ an avocado

zest of 2 lemons

⅓ cup lemon juice

1½ cups almond milk

2 tablespoons raw honey

pale, mild greens

Blend and top with grated lemon zest.

Orange Poppyseed Cake

  1 orange, peeled, segmented, and frozen

  zest and flesh of 1 orange, peeled

  2 tablespoons agave or honey

  2 tablespoons poppy seeds

  ½ an avocado

  1½ cups almond milk

  pale, mild greens

Blend all ingredients except the poppy seeds. Add the seeds and stir through on low speed, or stir in manually. Serve garnished with poppy seeds and grated orange zest.

Peach Melba

  2 to 3 large, ripe peaches

  1 teaspoon vanilla extract or half a vanilla pod

  1 cup Raw Vanilla Ice Cream (page 229)

  1 cup water (or ice if you want it thicker)

  pale, mild greens

Blend for 1 to 2 minutes.

  For Raspberry Sauce:

  1 cup raspberries

  2 tablespoons honey, agave, or maple syrup

  squeeze of lemon juice

Blend till well combined.

Gently stir the raspberry sauce through each glass of smoothie with a spoon so it creates contrast in the glass, and add plenty of extra sauce on the top! Use the raspberry sauce within 24 hours or freeze any remaining sauce in an ice cube tray.

Thank you to Adele McConnell from www.vegiehead.com for the following two delicious recipes.

Peanut-Butter Cup

2 frozen bananas, sliced

2 to 3 tablespoons peanut butter

1 tablespoon raw cacao powder

1 cup ice cubes

I cup sunflower seed or pumpkinseed milk

spinach

Blend and top with crushed peanuts. Use any nut butter if peanut is not available or preferred.

Choc-Mint Pattie

2 frozen bananas, sliced

2 tablespoons raw cacao powder

1 cup ice cubes

2 drops pure peppermint essential oil

2 tablespoons agave nectar

1½ cups almond milk

1 cup torn kale

Blend and top with grated raw mint chocolate.

Raw Vanilla Ice Cream

1½ cups cashews, soaked 4 hours

½ cups young Thai coconut flesh

2 cups young Thai coconut water

1 cup agave and/or maple syrup

2 whole vanilla pods, quartered

good pinch of salt

Blend all the ingredients until well combined and smooth. You may need to stop and scrape down the sides of the blender jug a few times. If it's too thick, add a little more liquid. Pour the cream into ice cube trays and freeze. Once frozen, pop them out and store in a labeled bag or container in the freezer to use as needed for adding decadence to smoothies. To serve as ice cream, refrigerate the cream and churn in an ice cream maker or process the frozen ice cream blocks in a high-speed blender till it reaches a soft ice cream consistency.

Super Green Ice Cream Variation: Make vanilla ice cream as above and add 2 tablespoons green powder, like Deep Green Alkaliser, Vital Greens, or barley grass powder, and/or matcha green tea powder as needed when blending.

Green Sorbet

3 cups (750 grams) orange segments and pineapple pieces

2 tablespoons sweetener, like xylitol, honey, maple syrup, or agave

1 cup (250 grams) almond milk

1 to 2 handfuls spinach

Ice cream maker version: Blend all ingredients like a smoothie for 1 to 2 minutes, then refrigerate or freeze for 1 hour. Add to the ice cream maker and churn according to the manufacturer's instructions for 30 to 40 minutes. Serve immediately.

Thermomix version: Freeze the almond milk into ice cubes. Cut the fruit into small pieces and freeze.

Add the spinach with ¼ cup of water and blend on speed 5 till pureed. Add three-quarters of the frozen milk and fruit, and the sweetener. Blend on speed 9 for 20 seconds. Add the remaining frozen milk and fruit, and with the aid of the spatula, blend on speed 9 for another 40 seconds, or until well combined and resembling sorbet. Serve immediately.

Instant Chai Spice Mix

2 tablespoons ground cinnamon

1 tablespoon ground ginger

1 tablespoon ground cardamom

1 teaspoon ground star anise

½ teaspoon ground cloves

¼ teaspoon ground black pepper

Mix and store in a glass jar. Whole spices (except ginger) can be used as well. Use equivalent amounts of whole spices and grind in a mortar and pestle or spice grinder

Nut and Seed Milks

Nut and seed milks can be made two ways. The short way is to blend nut butters with water for instant milk; the long way involves soaking nuts or seeds, blending them with water, and straining the contents to separate the fiber from the milk.

The longer soaking method is the healthiest option, and eating nuts and seeds after they have been soaked is kinder to our digestion and improves nutrient availability. Soaking helps to deactivate substances that are stopping the nut or seed from growing, particularly protease inhibitors (protease is an enzyme that helps break down protein). Soaking also aids the removal of anti-nutrients like phytates that can interfere with mineral absorption, although this is more of an issue with grains than nuts or seeds. When soaking grain foods for cooking, like rice and quinoa, the addition of an acidifier helps with the removal of phytates such as whey or lemon juice. For nuts and seeds, the addition of salt to the soaking water helps with the removal of the enzyme inhibitors.

There is no real consensus as to how long to soak nuts and seeds and some say not to bother soaking the very fatty nuts like macadamias. If you have the time, soak nuts from morning to evening, or overnight. I recommend only soaking cashews for about 4 hours as they can get a bit slimy, and be sure to use them right away, as they can go bad quickly. Other soaked nuts and seeds can be stored for a day in the fridge, however, I suggest using them as soon as possible, whether you choose to turn them into a milk or dehydrate them (in a food dehydrator at 118°F/48°C) or in an oven on the lowest setting with the door ajar, for up to 24 hours).

You can soak the following raw nuts and seeds to make milk: almonds, Brazil nuts, hazelnuts, sunflower seeds, pumpkinseeds, sesame seeds, macadamia nuts, pistachios, pine nuts, pecans, walnuts, peanuts, and cashews. Here are a few guidelines for making the best nut milks:

- Soak macadamias, cashews, pistachios, and pine nuts for 2 to 4 hours.
- Soak almonds, Brazil nuts, hazelnuts, sunflower seeds, pumpkinseeds, sesame seeds, pecans, walnuts, and peanuts overnight or all day with ½ teaspoon salt per cup of nuts or seeds.
- For hemp milk, don't soak the seeds; just blend the seeds straight into the water. Use 2 tablespoons to ½ cup seeds to 4 cups of water.
- Once soaked, drain and rinse the nuts or seeds very well.
- Combine 1 cup of nuts or seeds (dry weight) with 3 to 6 cups of water, depending how rich you like your milk and what your nut and seed budget is, and blend for 1 to 2 minutes on high speed.
- Strain the mixture though a nut milk bag or cheesecloth over a large bowl. You will need to massage the liquid out

of the fiber; it's messy but good fun! You can use the left-over fiber in other recipes such as raw or cooked veggie burgers to save waste, or try it as a face and body scrub.

- The milk will keep for a day or two in the fridge. If not using within 24 hours, I suggest freezing it into ice cube trays. Once frozen, pop them out and keep in a labeled freezer bag or container.

- You can flavor your nut and seed milks by adding cacao, sweetener, vanilla, and/or spices. If using a vanilla bean, slice the bean longways and chop in half, blending it with the nuts or seeds from the beginning.

- For the quick version of nut milk, simply blend a nut or seed butter into water at a ratio of 1 tablespoon to 1 cup of water. To add nut butter to a green smoothie, just add the nut butter straight into the smoothie in the correct ratio to the amount of water used in the recipe.

- Nut butters can be made at home raw or by lightly roasting or toasting the nuts or seeds first. If you have a heavy-duty blender like a Blendtec, Vitamix, or Thermomix, follow the instructions provided to make delicious butters like tahini, and nut spreads like almond, macadamia, and hazelnut.

Appendix

Bibliography

BOOKS

Alexander, Stephanie. *The Cook's Companion: The Complete Book of Ingredients and Recipes for the Australian Kitchen.* New York: Penguin, 2004.

Amsden, Matt. *RAWvolution: Gourmet Living Cuisine.* New York: HarperCollins, 2006.

Bisci, Dr. Fred. *Your Healthy Journey: Discovering Your Body's Full Potential.* Bisci Lifestyle Books, 2008.

Blereau, Jude. *Wholefood for Children: Nourishing Young Children with Whole and Organic Foods.* Sydney, Australia: Murdoch Books, 2010.

Boutenko, Victoria. *Green for Life.* Berkeley, CA: North Atlantic Books, 2010.

Boutenko, Victoria. *Green Smoothie Revolution: The Radical Leap Towards Natural Health.* Berkeley, CA: North Atlantic Books, 2009.

Bremmes, Lesley. *The Complete Book of Herbs: A Practical Guide to Growing and Using Herbs.* RD Press, 1988.

Campbell, T. Colin, and Thomas M. Campbell II. *The China Study: The Most Comprehensive Study of Nutrition Ever Conducted and the Startling Implications for Diet, Weight Loss, and Long-Term Health.* Dallas, TX: BenBella Books, 2004.

Cohen, Alissa. *Living on Live Food.* Cohen Publishing Company, 2004.

Cousens, Gabriel. *Rainbow Green Live-Food Cuisine.* Berkeley, CA: North Atlantic Books, 2003.

Daniel, Kaalya T. *The Whole Soy Story: The Dark Side of America's Favorite Health Food.* Washington, D.C.: New Trends, 2005.

Dowding, Charles. *Salad Leaves for All Seasons: Organic Growing from Pot to Pot.* Totnes, Devon, UK: Green Books, 2008.

Erasmus, Udo. *Fats That Heal, Fats That Kill: The Complete Guide to Fats, Oils, Cholesterol, and Human Health.* Summertown, TN: Alive Books, 2001.

Fallon, Sally. *Nourishing Traditions: The Cookbook That Challenges Politically Correct Nutrition and the Diet Dictocrats.* Washington, D.C.: New Trends, 2001.

Graham, Dr. Douglas N. *The 80/10/10 Diet: Balancing Your Health, Your Weight, and Your Life One Luscious Bite at a Time.* Key Largo, FL: FoodnSport, 2006.

Harris, Ben Charles. *Eat the Weeds.* Barre Publishers, 1995.

Hill, Fionna. *Microgreens: How to Grow Nature's Own Superfood.* Richmond Hill, Ontario, Canada: Firefly Books, 2010.

Holford, Patrick. *The Low-GL Diet Bible: The Perfect Way to Lose Weight, Gain Energy, and Improve Your Health.* London: Piatkus Books, 2009.

Holford, Patrick. *The New Optimum Nutrition Bible.* Berkeley, CA: The Crossing Press, 2004.

Howell, Dr. Edward. *Enzyme Nutrition, The Food Concept: Unlocking the Secrets of Eating Right for Health, Vitality, and Longevity.* New York: Avery, 1986.

Irving, David Gerow. *The Protein Myth: Significantly Reducing the Risk of Cancer, Heart Disease, Stroke, and Diabetes While Saving the Animals and the Planet.* Berkeley, CA: O-Books, 2011.

Kenney, Matthew, and Sarma Melngailis. *Raw Food/Real World: 100 Recipes to Get the Glow.* New York: HarperCollins, 2005.

Lantz, Dr. Sarah, *Chemical Free Kids: Raising Healthy Children in a Toxic World.* Budina, Queensland, Australia: Joshua Books, 2009.

McFarlane, Annette. *Organic Vegetable Gardening.* Sydney, Australia: ABC Books, 2006.

McKeith, Gillian. *Living Food for Health: 12 Natural Superfoods to Transform Your Health.* London: Piatkus Books, 2004.

Melngailis, Sarma. *Living Raw Food: Get the Glow with More Recipes from Pure Food and Wine.* New York: HarperCollins, 2009.

Meyerowitz, Steve. *Power Juices Super Drinks: Quick, Delicious Recipes to Prevent and Reverse Disease.* New York: Kensington Books, 2000.

Murray, Michael T., Joseph Pizzorno, and Lara Pizzorno. *The Encyclopaedia of Healing Foods.* London: Piatkus Books, 2008.

O'Meara, Cyndi. *Changing Habits Changing Lives: The Australian Way to Good Food, Better Health, and More Energy.* Camberwell, Victoria, Australia: Penguin, 2007.

Patenaude, Frédéric. *The Raw Secrets: The Raw Food Diet in the Real World.* Montreal, Canada: Fredericpatenaude.com, 2006.

Pollan, Michael. *In Defense of Food: An Eater's Manifesto.* New York: Penguin, 2009.

Robbins, John. *The Food Revolution: How Your Diet Can Help Save Your Life and Our World*. San Francisco: Conari Press, 2001.

Sellman, Sherrill. *Hormone Heresy: What Women Must Know About Their Hormones*. Tulsa, OK: Get Well International, 2000.

Soria, Cherie, Brenda Davis, and Vesanto Melina. *The Raw Revolution Diet*. Summertown, TN: Book Publishing Company, 2008.

Virtue, Doreen, and Jenny Ross. *The Art of Raw Living Food: Heal Yourself and the Planet with Eco-Delicious Cuisine*. Carlsbad, CA: Hay House, 2009.

Wigmore, Ann, and Lee Pattinson. *The Blending Book: Maximizing Natures Nutrients: How to Blend Fruits and Vegetables for Better Health*. New York: Avery, 1997.

Wolfe, David. *Eating For Beauty*. San Diego, CA: Sunfood, 2007.

Wolfe, David, *Superfoods: The Food and Medicine of the Future*. Berkeley, CA: North Atlantic Books, 2009.

Young, Robert O., and Shelley Redford Young. *The pH Miracle: Balance Your Diet, Reclaim Your Life*. New York: Warner, 1992.

WEBSITES

Dr. Duke's Phytochemical and Ethnobotanical Databases
www.ars-grin.gov/duke/plants.html

Nutrition data
www.nutritiondata.com

Oxygen Radical Absorbance Capacity ORAC) of Selected Foods, USDA, 2007
www.phytochemicals.info/list-orac-values.php

Toxic Agents in Plants (Cornell University)
www.ansci.cornell.edu/plants/toxicagents/index.html

The Ultimate GL Database
www.gl.patrickholford.interactiveprofiling.com

USDA Natural Nutrient Database
www.nal.usda.gov/fnic/foodcomp/search

The World's Healthiest Foods
www.whfoods.com

Resources

PRODUCTS

E3Live AFA Blue-Green Algae
United States: www.e3live.com
United Kingdom: www.detoxyourworld.com
Australia: www.e3live.com.au

In-Liven Fermented Probiotic Superfood, Berry Radical Anti-oxidant Superfood, Deep Green Alkaliser
www.onlinesales.miessence.com (worldwide)

Marine Phytoplankton
United States: Longevity Superfoods and UMAC Core brands
www.longevitywarehouse.com
United Kingdom: Oceans Alive brand
www.detoxyourworld.com
Australia: Oceans Alive brand
www.conscious-choice.com

RAW FOOD ONLINE SHOPS

United States
www.longevitywarehouse.com
www.oneluckyduck.com
www.therawfoodworld.com

Canada
www.rawnutrition.ca
www.trulyorganicfoods.com
www.realrawfood.com

United Kingdom
www.detoxyourworld.com
www.funkyraw.com
www.rawliving.eu

Australia
www.lovingearth.net
www.conscious-choice.com
www.raw-pleasure.com.au

Vitamix Blenders
Worldwide: www.vitamix.com

Blendtec Blenders
United States: www.blendtec.com

Thermomix Blenders
Canada: www.easycooking.ca
United Kingdom: www.ukthermomix.com
Australia and New Zealand: www.thermomix.com.au

Acknowledgments

To my mum, for inspiring my personal quest to never stop learning about food and health. The pile of books by my bedside is not unlike yours! To my husband, Ben, my rock, for your unwavering support. Thank you for never, ever doubting my ability and for accepting my crazy work hours and late nights writing. To all of my talented contributors in this book and on my website, I am sincerely grateful for your expertise and recipes. And to Victoria Boutenko—this book would not exist without your creation of the green smoothie.

About the Author

Kristine Miles is a health professional with over fifteen years' experience. She is passionate about life-long learning, plant-based nutrition, and living a low-toxic lifestyle. Her mission is to promote health and well-being by empowering others to lead lives free of chemicals and full of real, delicious food. Kristine works full time as a physiotherapist in private practice, is a part time cooking demonstrator, and blogs on www.kristinemiles.com and www.greensmoothiecommunity.com. She is happily married and lives on Phillip Island, Victoria, Australia.